Staying Home

A Caregiver's Guide to Making Your House Alzheimer's Safe

By

Derrick Grant

Staying Home: A Caregiver's Guide to Making Your House Alzheimer's Safe was written as an extension of *Elder Guru,* a website devoted to information for professionals working in aging services.

Visit **www.ElderGuru.com** to stay current on aging issues.

About the Author

Derrick Grant has worked as a Licensed Social Worker in a multi-level nursing home and as a social services manager at an Area Agency on Aging, overseeing information and referral, outreach, and an Alzheimer's caregiver support program. He has also worked as the Director of Adult Day Services in a designated Alzheimer's care center. He now administers ElderGuru.com and works on policy related to Medicaid.

The contents within this manual are intended to assist caregivers (spouses, adult children, paid caregivers, etc.) with making easy, low-cost changes to their homes to help ensure the safety of a resident with Alzheimer's disease or related dementia.

wise age
books

CONTENTS

Introduction
PREPARING FOR THE JOURNEY AHEAD

"You gain strength, courage, and confidence by every experience in which you really stop to look fear in the face. You must do the things which you think you cannot do."

- Eleanor Roosevelt

Caring for someone with dementia is one of the hardest adjustments a caregiver can make. This role will challenge you emotionally, mentally, socially, and physically. Although there are various forms of dementia, Alzheimer's is the most common and its onset can be unexpected. As a caregiver, you will need to adapt to your loved one's changing needs and protect them. In order to keep them safe, it's critical that you learn about the disease and the ways in which it influences behavior, personality, and overall mental functioning. This book is for those who provide in-home care for people with Alzheimer's disease or related disorders.

There are many things to consider when caring for an individual diagnosed with dementia or Alzheimer's. Many decisions will need to be made as the person changes and requires new methods of help in order to keep him or her safe and happy. Making these decisions typically falls on the persons closest to the one needing care, those most involved in everyday decision-making on behalf of their loved one. Once diagnosed, it's important to discuss details about the future.

Since Alzheimer's is progressive in nature, symptoms will worsen over time. Each case is unique. There are many factors that play a key role regarding the progression of this disease.

If you are reading this book, you have likely been considering the issues you may face and perhaps have even worked through some of them already. You have probably come to the realization that your loved one can no longer live alone safely without making some alterations to their current living environment, if they can live alone at all.

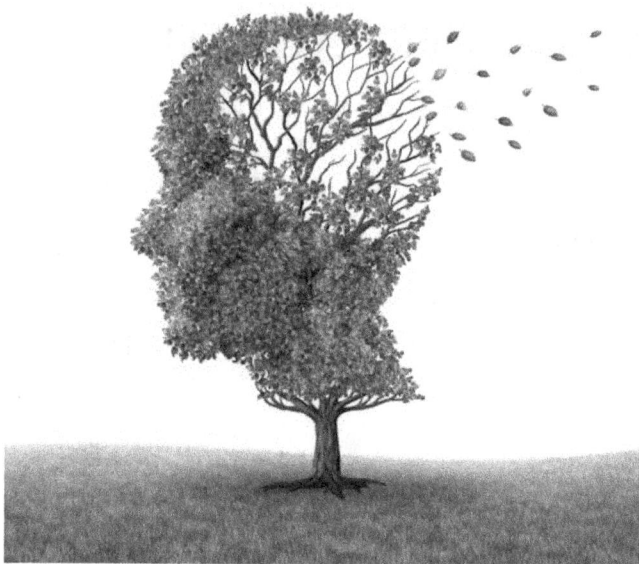

Watching your loved one's mind slip away may be the most difficult challenge you'll ever face.

Many of the suggestions in this manual can be used to alter the person's home so that they can stay independent longer or continue to live with their spouse or other family member. With that said, many of the suggested steps outlined here are made with the assumption that the person can no longer live alone. It is assumed that in the later stages, if they are not already, they will be moving in with someone who will act as a primary caregiver, someone who will tend to the person's daily needs.

The suggestions in this manual are intended to help you, as the caregiver, prepare your home. Once certain changes are made, you will be able to safely accommodate the person with Alzheimer's.

Meeting the individual's needs can be overwhelming as a caregiver, but there are ways to cope and overcome new challenges. Here are some tips for becoming familiar with your new role:

- **Arming yourself with knowledge about the disease is the first step when preparing to care for someone in need.** Becoming more educated will provide you with the tools and resources you require. Understanding how your loved one's abilities and personality will change will help you better prepare for the road ahead.

- **Having a support system is critical in helping to meet daily care needs for the individual.** These support systems are also instrumental in surviving the continual challenges as a caregiver. Support can come in many forms. The most obvious source of support comes from family and friends, but there are also support groups available, non-profit agencies that help seniors, and respite programs. These groups can be helpful to the caregiver in finding support, knowledge, and resources to deal with the ever-changing needs that occur when taking care of someone with Alzheimer's.

- **Preparing the physical home to accommodate the person with Alzheimer's will go a long way in helping ease the burden of caregiving.** Creating a simple environment that is easy to navigate will minimize fear and confusion, thus limiting the chance of increased agitation or aggression brought on by surroundings that are cluttered, unsafe, and confusing. A safe environment will also offer the caregiver greater peace of mind. This will reduce stress and worry surrounding potential accidents and physical injury.

- **If there are choices for your loved one to make, make them easy ones.** Having too many choices causes confusion in the person with Alzheimer's. Being able to make a choice—perhaps between just two things, such as which shirt to wear, will help your loved one maintain a positive sense of independence and well-being.

- **Make changes slowly.** Limit changes to only those that are necessary at that time, unless planning ahead (remodeling, for example) is required. Too many changes all at once could cause confusion. Going slowly will also make the tasks easier and may prevent making changes that may never be needed.

When you effectively prepare your home in order to meet the needs of someone with Alzheimer's, you will:

- Minimize fear and confusion
- Reduce the risk of injury
- Promote caregiver ease and reduce overall stress
- Create a more comfortable environment

As you go through this manual and look at the living environment you're planning to make safe, consider what will work in your particular situation. Many of the alterations discussed in this book are inexpensive and easy to implement. Other changes that require hiring help or buying expensive equipment will naturally cost more.

Whatever you do, make a plan. Walk through your house and make notes based on potential hazards in each room. What will restrict good care? What could pose a danger? After you look at the inside of the house, go outside to look at your yard and other outdoor areas. There will likely be a lot of potential hazards outdoors that you will have to be addressed in order to make it safe for your loved one to enjoy the outside.

First look at what changes you can implement fairly easily. Consider where your loved one is in the disease process and how much extra assistance is needed, as well as what's affordable. Cost is a major consideration for many homeowners.

Depending on your loved one's immediate needs, implement the cheapest safety options first. As your budget allows for greater alterations, match new changes to your loved one's changing needs. If your budget is tight, prioritize in terms of the most critical changes. Is your loved one wandering often, trying to leave the home? In this case, installing an effective lock system or alarm will be important.

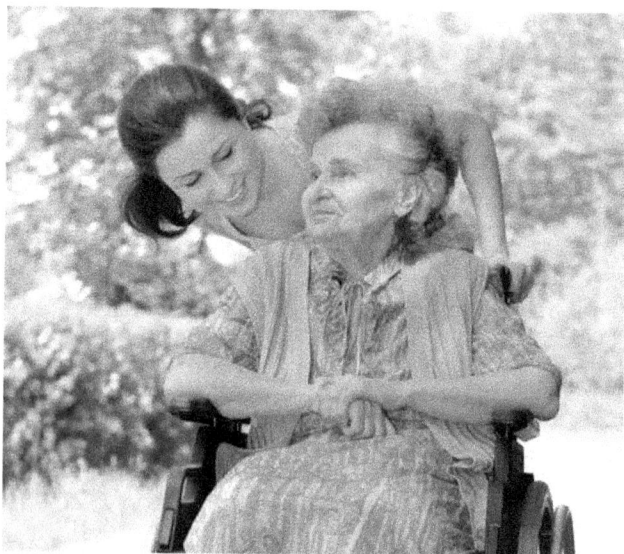

Ensuring safety outdoors is essential, as your loved one will highly benefit from fresh air and sunlight. This is especially true regarding their sleep-wake cycle, as disrupted sleeping patterns are generally an area of concern for people with Alzheimer's. Spending time outdoors will also reduce their risk of a Vitamin D deficiency.

This manual will help you address each room, based on your personal circumstances. The suggestions here should make you more aware of what dangers lie in your own home and what should be changed to avert potential injury or—at minimum—confusion and fear.

If you are a parent, you will see that addressing issues in the home is similar to preparing a safe environment for a small, curious child. The child may not know safety from harm. The child will touch and ingest things they shouldn't. There is a crucial difference, however. The home you're preparing is not for a child, but for a confused adult with years of life experience.

We will consider each room of your house then move to the garage and exterior areas. Many of the items and tools you will need can be found in your local department or hardware stores. Other items can be found at specialty stores and online.

The main hope and objective is to offer you the information, support, and resources required when making your home safer. In turn, you will feel more comfortable and secure as you continue to care for your loved one. Dealing with Alzheimer's is not easy for anyone—for the individual, the caregiver, and even for professionals. Having everything possible at your disposal in terms of information and support will help you along this journey.

Once you or a loved one has been diagnosed with Alzheimer's, it is tough for everyone involved. Although it's important to take the time to grieve and stabilize emotions, planning for the future is essential. In order to avoid tough decisions in future years, speaking with the individual affected regarding their wishes is important during the early stages. As their disease progresses, those closest to the individual will need to continually make tough daily decisions.

In the beginning, the decisions are generally focused around what to do next. This can be overwhelming for a caregiver, but there are specific steps that one should take to start on the right track. Go see the person's physician. Get to know him or her so that you are able to ask questions and gain support.
Each time you notice changes in your loved one's ability or behavior, write them down. It's important to keep your loved one's physician in the loop. They're not with them on a daily basis like you are. This can help shape their personal treatment plan. Although there isn't a cure for Alzheimer's, there are ways to reduce certain symptoms while enhancing their overall quality of life.

Many former assumptions should be questioned as the person diagnosed with Alzheimer's becomes less able to do the things he or she formerly could. Does the individual still have a job? Can he or she still go to work and perform those duties? Is the person safe to drive? A big question is whether the person diagnosed with Alzheimer's is even able to continue to live within their current living situation, and if they are, how long they will be able to.

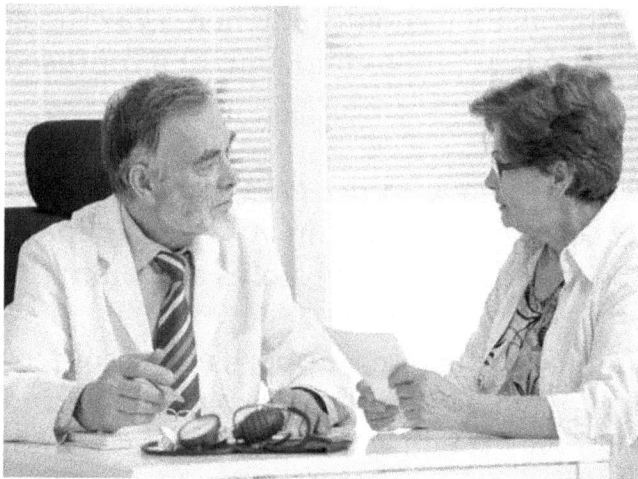

When you develop a relationship with your loved one's physician, you will have access to information and advice that can help you make more informed decisions.

This manual will help you better understand your loved one's condition while ensuring their safety. You are probably aware of what caregiving needs you will be facing. You may have watched for many years as your loved one has developed this illness. You are aware of the memory issues, the oncoming depression, and the bouts of agitation and anger that can emerge. You have seen physical and emotional needs change. You are preparing to overcome these challenges to help cope with any changes your loved one will continue to face.

Not only will you need to make changes to your home, but there are various mental and emotional needs to consider. Changes in cognition and understanding will have a profound effect on how your loved one copes with daily life. He or she will no longer be able to do the daily tasks that many people take for granted—paying bills, driving a car, even following a recipe. The person affected with dementia or Alzheimer's may no longer understand things you tell him. They may see things that are not there or believe things that are not true, and you will not be able to convince him or her otherwise; you will just have to deal with the fact that they believe what they believe. This is referred to as "meeting them where they are." Trying to correct the person's reality can often cause anxiety.

As one's cognition diminishes, you will notice changes in their physical abilities, level of functioning, and overall behavior. Individuals may pace the floor, wander, or become increasingly restless. Sleep patterns will surely change as sleeplessness may occur at night, with frequent trips to the bathroom. They may also get up in the middle of the night without purpose.

All of these changes are confusing to deal with. Knowing that they exist and learning how to deal with them will help provide a safe and secure environment.

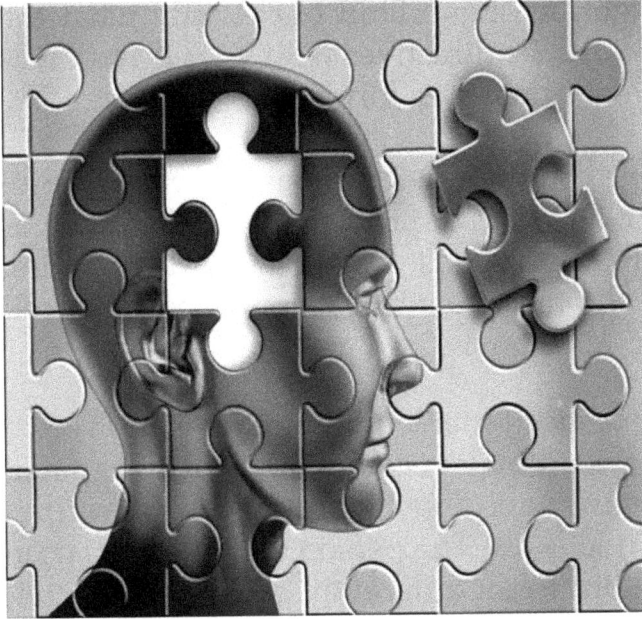

It's crucial to acknowledge that Alzheimer's is a progressive disease that directly impacts the brain.

WHAT TO EXPECT

"When people say, 'You have Alzheimer's,' you have no idea what Alzheimer's is. You know it's not good. You know there's no light at the end of the tunnel. That's the only way you can go. But you really don't know anything about it. And you don't know what to expect."

- Nancy Reagan

In the beginning, when faced with the often frightening diagnosis of Alzheimer's, everything can seem overwhelming. If your loved one hasn't included you in the

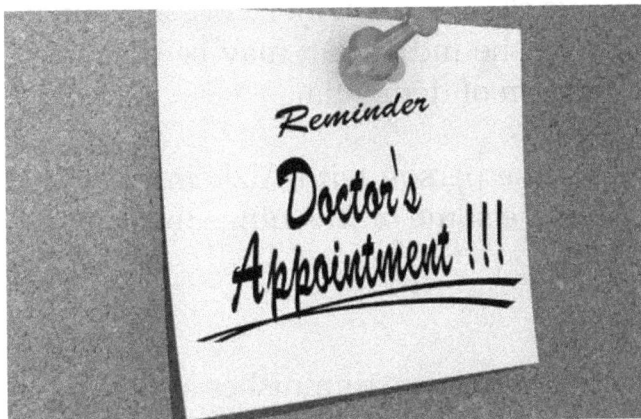

Going to your loved one's appointments is imperative. Keep notes on changes and address any concerns at each appointment.

doctor's visits up until now, it's time to get involved. Find out exactly what the doctor is saying. Discuss the need for any advance directives with your loved one's doctor. This includes living wills and powers of attorney forms.

As mentioned, Alzheimer's is a progressive condition with no known cure. Symptoms can only be managed. The first sign of any kind of problem generally involves memory, with incidents noticed by family and friends. Dad may start forgetting where he puts the keys (more often than the rest of us do). Mom repeats herself more, or she forgets the grandkids' names.

You may have noticed other changes—a once well-manicured mother is now often unkempt, with messy hair or dirty clothes. Dad may become more easily agitated when the grandchildren are noisy. Mom may not be able to create the great recipes she once did. Judgment is skewed. Perception is off. The person with dementia can no longer cover their shortcomings and begins to act differently. All of these inconsistencies begin to add up until the people around realize that something is wrong.

People with dementia experience loss of short-term memory, along with other cognitive issues such as diminished judgment and poor planning.

According to the Alzheimer's Association, *dementia is a condition in which a person has significant difficulty with daily functioning because of problems with thinking and memory. Dementia is not a single disease. It's an overall term — like 'heart disease' — that* covers a wide range of specific medical conditions, including Alzheimer's disease. A classic example of this is vascular dementia, which often develops after an individual has a stroke. Within Alzheimer's disease, there are clear hallmarks in the form of proteins, known as plaques and tangles. In turn, areas of the brain become damaged.

As behaviors change, the person affected will appear very different to those close to him or her. When two or more of these cognitive changes—memory loss accompanied with another—are present, there is a chance the individual may be diagnosed with Alzheimer's, as this is the most common form of dementia.

What kinds of things should be expected from the person with Alzheimer's? That depends on the stage of one's disease, but here are some of the things that you can expect:

- Forgetting familiar people and places
- Requiring more and more support, as independence diminishes

- Possible aggressive behavior
- Increased confusion
- Wandering
- Poor sleep patterns

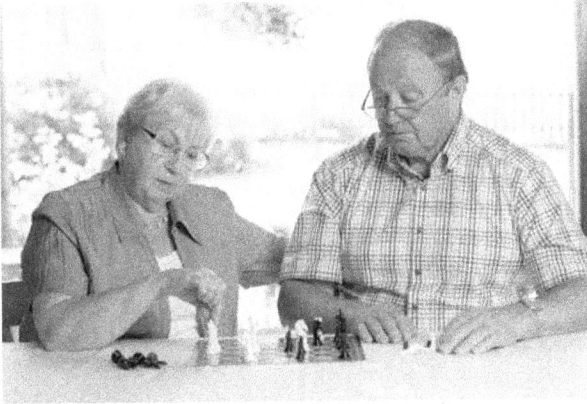

Patience and understanding will help both the caregiver and the loved one as the disease progresses.

Changes and understanding will be required. It may confuse loved ones when Grandpa can't remember the kids' names but remembers the year he received his diploma from college. He may remember his own mother, who died long ago, but doesn't recognize his own daughter. He may even think his daughter *is* his mother. When it comes to Alzheimer's, long-term memory may remain intact to some extent until the end of life, while short-term memory is significantly hindered. The person with Alzheimer's usually knows, at least in the early stages of the disease, that something is not right. Individuals are often aware that they forget things they shouldn't, or that they cannot do the things they used to. As the disease progresses, many will retreat to an earlier time in their mind, when they lived as a young adult or child. Do not try to reorient the individual to the present. This can increase confusion. Listen to and understand the individual. Encourage him or her to recall the memories. If they enjoy them, surround the person with photographs and music from that time. Dealing with these losses can cause fear in a person as he or she does not completely understand what is happening. Embarrassment is also a natural feeling, as the person is no longer able to figure out how to do tasks that should be simple.

It's important to note that each individual's case is unique. There are many factors involved in the onset and progression of one's condition. The greatest variation of symptoms will be apparent within the earliest stages, as some still maintain an impressive degree of independence while others deteriorate rapidly.

As the individual's condition progresses, more and more common symptoms will surface. Individuals with dementia may experience paranoia, delusions, and hallucinations. A common paranoid delusion in those with dementia is that someone—maybe even a family member—is stealing from them. This is because they forget where they put things. They may even see or hear things that aren't there.

When this happens, all the caregiver can do is listen. Validate their feelings instead of trying to convince them of something else. In other words, "meet them where they are." The worst thing you can do is argue. This will only cause distress for both of you.

Always remember, your loved one is not being difficult on purpose. The individual may become fearful of people or everyday activities. One common fear among those with dementia is bathing. Whether they feel it's an invasion of privacy or the environment is too cold, resisting help with bathing is common.

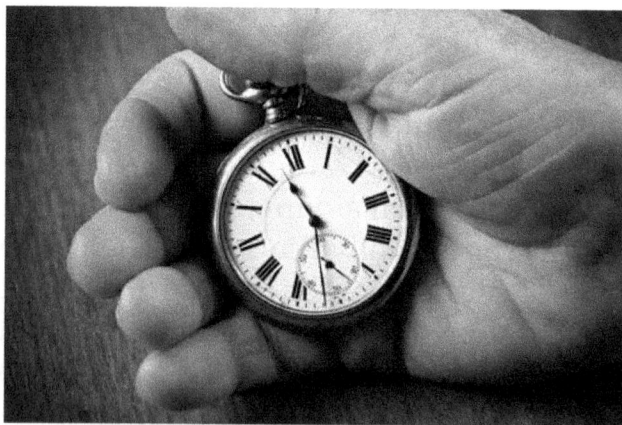

Your loved one's mood may change with the time of day, particularly at night.

Depression also accompanies dementia. All of these symptoms that arise should be discussed with the physician. There are medications that can help manage symp-toms. It's also critical that you encourage them to consume a healthy diet and to stay active. This will also help reduce symptoms of depression and anxiety.

One of the most difficult behaviors to manage is called sundowning. It gets its name because it is timed with the setting of the sun. Sundowning is a common behav-ior among those with Alzheimer's. Late in the afternoon and early in evening, the person may exhibit increased confusion and agitation. He or she may be restless, wandering more than usual, looking for someone or something. They may be more aggressive, whether verbally or physically. One theory is that it is the time of day when a person may feel like they should leave work to go home or get the kids, causing anxiety that they feel they should do *something*, but they don't know what. Again, this type of behavior should be discussed with a physician.

Knowing that sundowning is a normal part of the disease helps the caregiver accept the behaviors that may occur. Medications can help, but it is best to try identifying the cause of any confusion. Perhaps there are direct changes that can be made to make the individual more relaxed.

Managing an individual's surroundings is an important aspect in managing dementia. Keep in mind that there are no fixed answers. As the disease progresses and the person continues to change, the environment may have to change with them. What works for one person may not work for another. That's why it is important that you:

- Try different things to see what works and what doesn't
- Talk to others who are going through the same thing
- Contact your loved one's doctor or other professionals who specializes in dementia
- Involve family members
- Get support for yourself as caregiver

You can't take care of another without first taking care of yourself. Taking care of yourself and your surroundings will help to make life more manageable for both of you. You'll be both taking care of yourself and your loved one if you make your job easier. Connect with others by reaching out to the Alzheimer's Association in your state, your local Area Agency on Aging, and similar organizations. A list of these resources can be found by visiting **www.ElderGuru.com**. Of course, your job will be made easier by making sure your living environment is made as safe as it can be.

CHAPTER ONE
GUIDELINES FOR THE ENTIRE HOME

We will go through the main rooms of the house, as well as the exterior, from the front door throughout the safety of the fenced-in yard, but we will start with general guidelines for the entire home. If you follow the suggestions outlined in this manual, you are off to an excellent start, ensuring safe surroundings for the person with dementia who is in your care. Think about your preparations similarly to child-proofing your home. Think prevention first and foremost. Then remove or make alterations on anything that could be dangerous.

GENERAL GUIDELINES

- **Display emergency numbers and your home address near all telephones.**

- **Use an answering machine when you cannot answer phone calls.** Set it to turn on after the fewest number of rings possible. A person with Alzheimer's disease may be unable to take messages or could become victim of telephone exploitation. Turn ringers on low to avoid distraction and confusion.

- **Remove any items that might be dangerous.** Put away the ironing board, or at least lock away the iron. Lock up curling irons and space heaters. Any small appliances that can be plugged in should be locked away out of sight.

- **Electrical outlets should be plugged with child-safety caps or plate covers.**

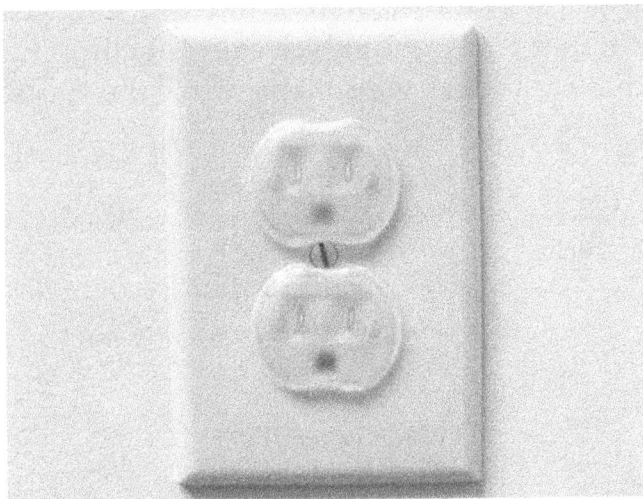

Many items sold for infant safety can also be used for Alzheimer's, like these plugs that cover electrical outlets.

- **Look for any item that could be used as a weapon and cause harm.** Put away sharp objects such as scissors, letter openers, and tweezers. Check your bathroom counters and accessible drawers for these types of objects. Check cabinets and drawers in every room to ensure that all sharp objects are removed.

- **Remember to check every room for houseplants that could be eaten and could cause illness or worse.** Artificial plants could be tempting, too, and should be removed if they become a problem.

- **Look at locks throughout the house.** Only have locks on interior doors that you plan to have off-limits. The loved one's bedroom, the bathroom, and other allowed areas should not have locks on them. Make sure locks on exterior doors are out of reach or too difficult to figure out how to unlock.

- **Choose appropriate locks for different types of windows.**

- **Put child safety locks on cabinets as needed.**

- **Put a cover on the thermostat.**

- **It might be prudent to lock up dangerous items in any off-limits rooms just in case a door is left unlocked or the person somehow finds his or her way to that normally forbidden room.** Examples include scissors in the sewing room and gasoline in the garage.

- **Stairs inside the house are an obvious danger.** Make sure there is at least one handrail that extends beyond the first and last steps. Consider painting contrasting colors to distinguish the steps. Handrails are a must. If the area must be blocked off, do so with a gate that is tall enough to prevent climbing over it. Safety gates should be placed at the foot as well as the top of the stairs.

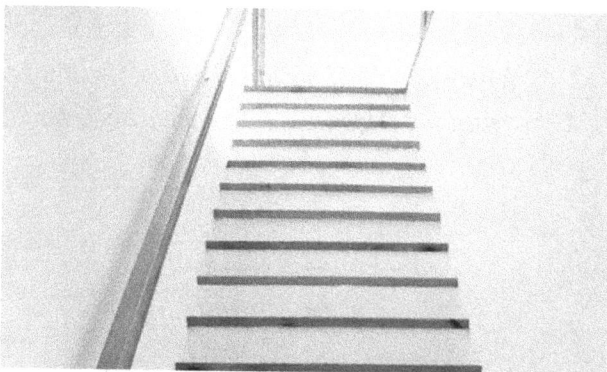

The contrast between the wood steps and the white risers makes each step easy to see.

- **Go through the house to see if colors have been chosen to aid in getting around.** Look at the contrast of floors next to the walls, as well as the walls to the curtains. Is the furniture easy to spot, as it provides a contrast to the floor beneath? This is especially important in being able to find a comfortable chair quickly.

- **Look at lighting in each room.** Make sure that there is plenty of overhead lighting in each room, paying special attention to the areas where the person will be dressing, bathing, and conducting other activities of daily living. This includes the bedroom, the bathroom, the shower, and any vanity area. Look at the lighting at different times of the day. Lighting that casts shadows on walls can be scary to the person with dementia. Add night lights everywhere needed.

- **Check all the doorways to make sure they are wide enough.** Feel around the frame for smooth edges. Are doorknobs easy to turn? If not, consider replacing them with levers to provide easier access. For the rooms that are shut off, cover doorknobs or lock these rooms.

- **Install smoke alarms and carbon monoxide detectors in or near the kitchen and all sleeping areas.** Check batteries often. Place fire extinguishers in key places.

- **Hide a spare key outside.** Your loved one may accidentally lock you out of the house.

- **If smoking is permitted, monitor the person with Alzheimer's while he or she is smoking.** Remove matches, lighters, ashtrays, cigarettes, and other means of smoking from view. This reduces fire hazards, and with these reminders out of sight, the person may forget the desire to smoke.

- **Keep plastic bags out of reach.** A person with Alzheimer's disease may choke or suffocate if plastic bags are used inappropriately.

- **Remove all guns and other weapons from the home or luck them up.** If kept in the home, as a second safety measure, add safety locks to the guns, remove firing pins, and secure ammunition in a separate location.

- **Restrict access to the computer and Internet.** Protect important files with passwords and back those files up. Consider monitoring computer use by the person with Alzheimer's, and install software that screens for objectionable material on the Internet.

Ensure that the person with dementia has plenty of room to walk around the house, wandering within rooms and between rooms. Take a walk yourself throughout the house. Are pathways clear? Do you have to maneuver to get around pieces of furniture?

Is there a danger of running into the pictures on the wall? Move whatever is in the way to ensure safe movement from room to room. Remember to allow wider spaces for walkers and wheelchairs or place chairs in strategic areas to provide rest areas.

ROOMS TO CONSIDER MAKING OFF-LIMITS

The Laundry Room

- **Washers and dryers can be turned on, misused, and have inappropriate items stuck in them.**

- **Wandering hands can get into laundry detergent, softener, and even bleach.** The laundry room likely holds numerous chemicals that could be toxic if swallowed.

- **If the laundry area is simply a closet, close it off with a child-proof lock.** If it's not possible to shut off the laundry room because it's a part of the bathroom or other area, then make sure that any chemicals are locked up in the cabinets.

- **Unplug the washer and dryer when not in use.** Always check to see if anything has been stuffed in either appliance before dumping in clothes and turning on the power.

The Personal Office

- **Look at the expensive equipment that is in this space, including items**

such as a computer, a printer, a fax machine. These costly electronics may be tempting to work with or susceptible to being knocked off the desk or table.

- **Filing cabinets provide opportunities for pilfering through important files and even losing them.**

- **Bookcases may pose as a climbing temptation.**

- **Various supplies could be dangerous.**

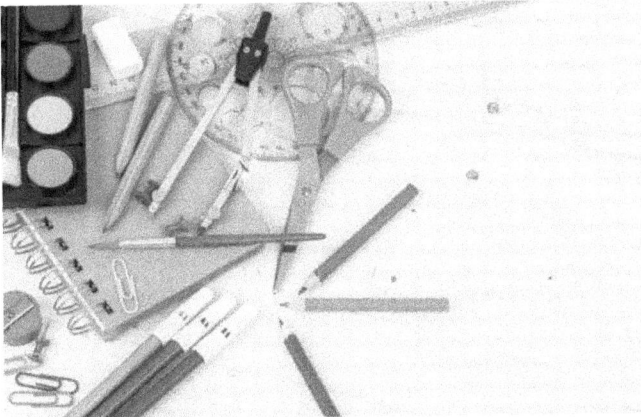

Go through your home and say to yourself, "Could this item cause harm to my loved one?"

Due to the dangers in the room, simply locking the door will ensure that your equipment and your loved one stay safe.

Sewing and Craft Rooms

- **Besides the obvious danger of a sewing machine, there are scissors and needles, strings and threads, and small items such as buttons.** Items can be lost, chewed on, and even swallowed.

- **If the person with dementia has a place to sit and visit with the person working in the room, then supervised visits in that room may be fine.** When not in use, however, it is best to deny access.

The Garage

- **Keep the door to the garage locked at all times.** Go a step further and hide car keys to avoid any temptation to get into the car or upset feelings when that desire is denied.

- **Many garages hold lawn equipment, including lawn mowers and weed eaters, which definitely should be kept off limits.**

- **Garages sometimes have inviting work areas and lots of tools.** They house sharp could-be weapons, such as shovels, axes, hoes, and rakes. Garages also store oil, paint, and other chemicals that could be deadly if ingested.

- **If access to the garage is granted, lock all power tools and machinery.**

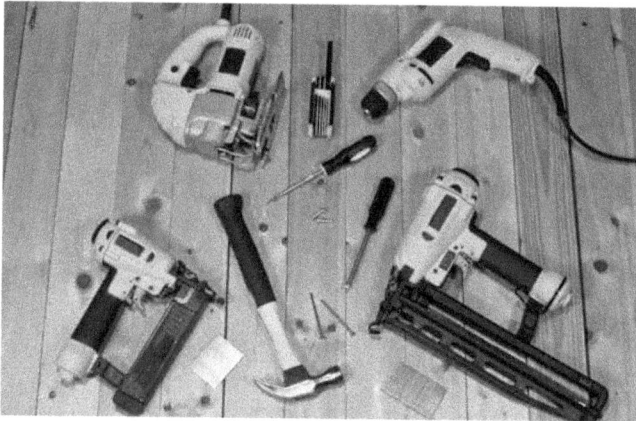

Garages and workshops may harbor many items that are no longer safe for your loved one to use.

A final thing to think about are the pets in the home. Homes with pets must make adjustments to ensure safety for both the person and the pets. It is entirely possible that the person with dementia might eat cat or dog food, or mess with the litter box. For this reason, put these items in out-of-the-way places, such as the off-limits laundry room. You may have to install a doggy door to allow free access for dogs to their food or cats to the litter box.

Keep fish tanks out of reach. The combination of glass, water, electrical pumps, and potentially poisonous aquatic life could be harmful to a curious person with Alzheimer's disease.

You may have other areas that are specific to your own house or living arrangements that you will need to check and adjust to make as safe as possible. After going through this manual, you will most likely be able to see areas in a way you hadn't before and adjust accordingly.

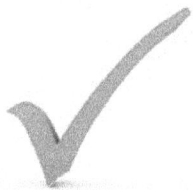

CHAPTER ONE CHECKLIST

____I have displayed emergency numbers and the home address near all telephones.

____I have set an answering machine to answer calls when I cannot. I have set it to turn on after the fewest number of rings possible.

____I have removed any items that might be dangers: clothes iron, space heaters, alcohol, etc.

____I have installed child-safety caps or plate covers over electrical outlets.

____I have put away sharp objects such as scissors, letter openers, tweezers, etc.

____ I have checked every room for houseplants that could be eaten and cause illness.

____I have chosen appropriate locks for different types of windows and cabinets.

____I have covered the thermostat.
____I have installed smoke alarms and carbon monoxide detectors in or near the kitchen and all sleeping areas.

____I have hidden a spare house key outside in case my loved one accidentally locks me out of the house.
____I have removed or secured all guns or other weapons.

____I have restricted access to the computer and Internet or set appropriate software to screen for objectionable material.

CHAPTER TWO
THE BEDROOM

We need to address each room in the house and there's no doubt that the bedroom is one of the most important rooms to start with. The bedroom is where people spend much of their time, resting, sleeping, and dressing. When you take the proper steps, the bedroom may also act as a haven or get-away for someone with dementia. This could be their special space, a place to read, to do crossword puzzles, or even rummage through his or her personal items. There are a number of adjustments, many of them simple, which can be implemented to ensure a safe and comfortable bedroom retreat.

STEP ONE: MAKE SURE IT IS WELL-LIT

People with dementia may suffer from changing vision and a well-lit room can make a big difference in their ability to get around. Ask yourself these questions:

- Is the light switch easy to find?
- Is the wattage bright enough?
- Is there a light source beside the bed?

Equip overhead light fixtures with the highest wattage they will handle. To help find the light switch in a dim room, you can purchase and install brightly covered light switches or even switch plates that glow in the dark.

Consider removing lamps entirely as they are harder to turn on and off. Eliminating lamps will reduce the risks of touching hot bulbs or tripping over cords. Fumbling for a lamp switch also makes it easy to knock lamps off tables, resulting in broken glass and feelings of failure.

In addition to adequate overhead lighting, one or two nightlights that come on automatically when the room darkens are strongly encouraged. If getting up to go to the bathroom at night occurs—and chances are it will, these nightlights will become a necessity.

There are now even nightlights that sit atop nightstands and glow from below. *Blys* produces such a light that provides a low-level glow, allowing uninterrupted sleep, but on waking provides a focus in the room while illuminating important items on top of it: water, phone, glasses, etc. These speciality products can be pricey, though, from $170-$200.

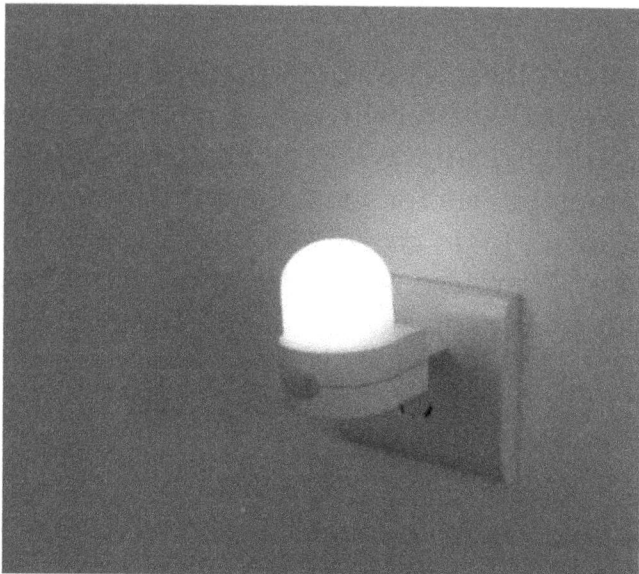

Low-cost and useful, night lights should be added to every room.

STEP TWO: ASSESS WALL COLORS

New caregivers are often surprised at this suggestion. Changing wall colors is not something most people would think of, but wall color can make a big difference in being able to get around the room and find things. The colors of the walls and furnishings affect mood. Bright, warm colors such as yellow or peach provide mood support as well as more light in the room. Light blue and gray colors may be hard to see and should be avoided. Dark colors will obviously darken the room and should not be used. Contrasting colors between the wall and the floor will help the individual's depth perception.

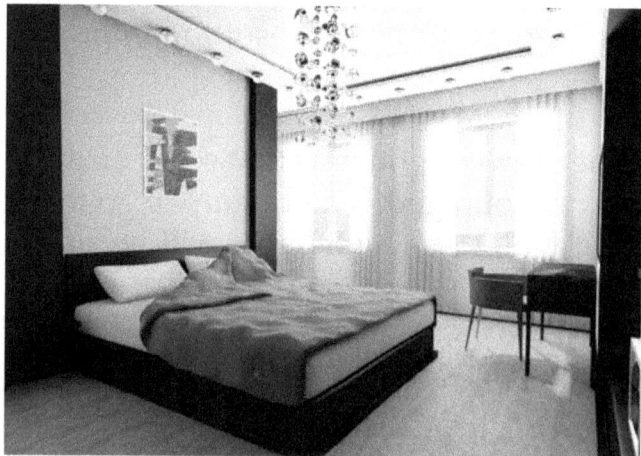

Contrasting colors between bed, floor, and walls will make a room much easier to navigate.

Too many colors or prints, whether on the walls or throughout the room, are distracting and can cause confusion and anxiety. Simple is good.

Step Three: Make It Safe

Make getting around the room easier by eliminating clutter and tripping hazards. Remove unnecessary furnishings and furniture that are in the way and could increase the risk of accidents. Create an easy-to-follow pathway from the bed to the bathroom or bedroom door. Trash cans aren't only a potential tripping hazard. As the disease progresses, they can be seen as a toilet. Removing trashcans from the bedroom may be a wise idea.

Add a chair if there isn't one. This will allow the individual to rest, read, and relax. Besides removing breakable lamps, take out any breakable or sharp-edged decorations. Look for anything that someone could trip on, and get it out of the room.

Remove mirrors. The person with dementia is often confused by who they see in the mirror. Reduce anxiety by removing them.

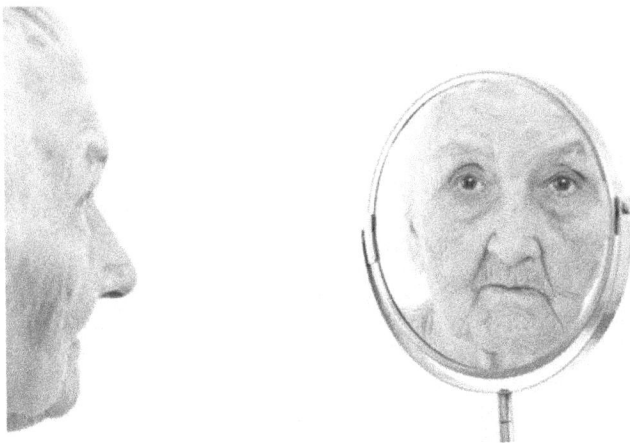

Your loved one may think he or she is younger than she is, causing confusion when they look in the mirror.

Look at the furniture in the bedroom. What might be dangerous? Ask yourself:

- Should I change dressers or other items with sharp edges, or put padding on the corners?
- Is the nightstand wobbly?
- Does the side table have a glass top?
- Is the furniture sturdy enough to lend support if someone leans on it?
- Are curtains flame-retardant? Are the patterns too busy?

STEP FOUR: SIMPLIFY

Remember, individuals with Alzheimer's and dementia become easily confused. To make things less overwhelming, it's important to simplify their living space. Here are a few tips so that you can make immediate changes:

- **Eliminate clutter in the closet**. You can install an automatic light that comes on when the closet door is opened and goes off when the door is closed. If the closet doors are difficult to maneuver, remove them and install a light that is motion-activated. These motion sensor lights can cost as little as $10.

- **Organize the closet with a small number of hanging clothes.** Offer the individual choices, but not so many choices that they are easily overwhelmed. Make sure everything is within reach to prevent falling. Keep shoes off the floor and placed in holders that can be easily seen and reached.

- **Simplify clothing choices in dressers.** Label drawers to keep your loved more independent in dressing themselves for as long as possible. Use words or pictures on labels. Again, present choices, but not too many choices.

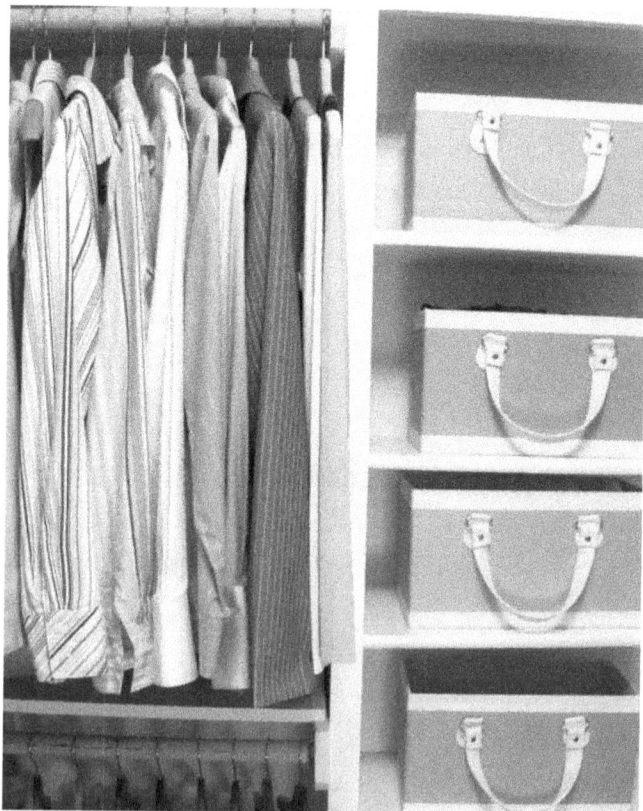

A well-organized closet makes it easier to remain independent with dressing.

- **Remove unnecessary items or items with sharp edges**.

- **Consider filling some drawers with personal items appropriate for rummaging**. This activity can be a great way to pass time. Having drawers for just this purpose will prevent some unwanted plundering through items in other rooms. Fill the drawers with items of interest, such as scarves, handkerchiefs, a wallet, and old photos.

STEP FIVE: ENSURE A COMFORTABLE TEMPERATURE

As your loved one may spend a lot of time in the bedroom, a comfortable temperature will be essential. That temperature may be warmer than what the rest of the home's inhabitants might prefer, so it may be necessary to close vents in the other rooms. Avoid using a space heater unless you plan to keep a very close eye on your loved one. A space heater could be knocked over, tripped on, or generally present a fire hazard.

STEP SIX: ASSESS THE BED

Take a good look at the bed. It is important to have a safe, comfortable bed that one can get easily in and out of. Using your loved one's own bed for as long as possible will make him feel more at home. Here are a few tips to ensure comfort and safety:

- **Make sure the sleeping area is easy to identify**. Use bedding with colors that contrast with the colors of the walls and floor.

- **The mattress should be firm and supportive**. It is recommended that it be protected with a waterproof cover in order to protect it from any incontinence. It never hurts to have a fire retardant mattress and bedding, either.

- **You may need to raise the bed with risers to make it easier to get in and out of.** These can be purchased through most department stores for as little as $10. On the other hand, if your loved one is prone to falls, lowering the height may be what needs to be done. You may have to get rid of the frame to make the bed low enough.

- **Hard bedframes with sharp corners should be replaced.** To help cushion any falls from the bed, you can place a soft mat or pillows on the floor beside it. With a low bed and a soft mat on the floor, the chance of injury should be small.

- **Consider bed placement**. You might place one side of the bed against the wall to lessen the chances of rolling off the bed. There are two sides to this. Having the bed against the wall also limits access and as care needs progress, the bed may need to be moved out from the wall in order to care for the person from either side.

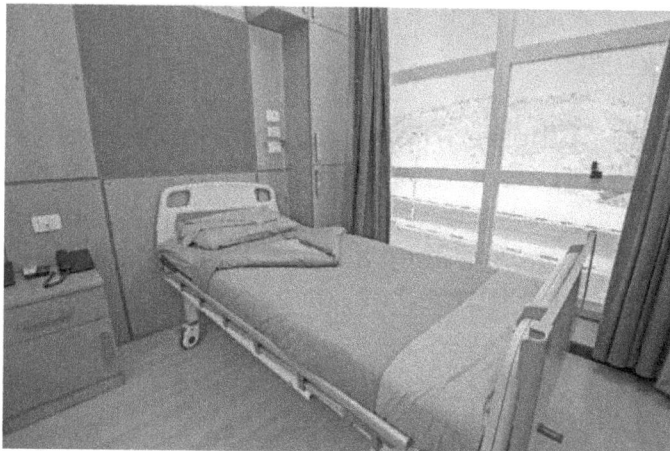

A hospital bed that raises and lowers could be a big help as mobility decreases.

- **Beware of bed rails.** Some people believe that bed rails are the answer to keeping one safely in the bed. Not true! Raised rails frequently prove to be more of a danger. The person with dementia may try to climb over them, resulting in injury, or get an arm stuck in them. A low bed and mat on the floor are a safer option.

- **Bed bars, similar to grab bars, can be installed near the bed to help the person pull himself or herself out of the bed**. If you do opt for some type of bar near the bed, purchase accompanying padding to soften it.

- **A "hospital bed" may eventually be needed.** This type of bed has controls that can lift either end of the bed up or down and is often covered by Medicare and other insurance plans.

If the level of care exceeds what you can physically do, remember that there is help out there. If you can no longer lift or help transfer your loved one out of the bed and into a chair, there is equipment to help with that, too. Visit the resources section of this book to connect with agencies that can further assist. Don't risk hurting yourself or your loved one.

STEP SEVEN: REDUCE THE RISK OF FALLS

Although bed bars are great, there are other options to ensure safety. Preventing falls is important as injuries can be significant. Other ways to reduce the chance of a fall include:

- **A pressure sensitive pad can be placed under the bedding without compromising comfort.** Significant movements will alert the caregiver — hopefully in time to prevent a fall. Similar devices can be attached to a chair, giving the same kind of warning. These devices can be very helpful in preventing injuries and cost typically $50-$75.

- ***Don't* put heating pads or electric blankets on beds or chairs.** People with dementia won't recognize when their skin is getting too hot from the heat and they may not know how to turn off the power.

- **Make sure the carpeting is secure and doesn't pose a trip hazard.** Use adhesive backings for mats or throw rugs, or remove them completely. Avoid high gloss cleaning agents on hardwood floors. Individuals with dementia are often frightened by freshly waxed, shiny floors, as they look slippery.

STEP EIGHT: MAKE AN EASY PATH FROM BEDROOM TO BATHROOM

Getting up in the middle of the night can be confusing for someone with dementia. If a bathroom is located in the bedroom, install nightlights along the path to the bathroom. This will reduce fear and anxiety while reducing the risk of tripping. Other suggestions:

- **Make sure the person can first find the door exit the bedroom.** You can accomplish this by painting the door a different color or even just the door frame. If the bathroom is down the hall, put nightlights in the hallway, along with handrails to help guide the person to the bathroom. If needed, label the bathroom with a bright or glow-in-the-dark sign.

- **Consider adult pads for night use.** If getting up at night results in injury, particularly if the person has incontinence issues, it might be time for adult pads. There are high-quality pads and adult diapers on the market that hold moisture, such as urine, away from the skin to prevent skin rash and breakdown. Use of these items could help prevent injuries at night while helping ensure a good night's sleep for the person with dementia.

- **Help your loved one attend to any toileting needs right before bedtime to reduce the need to get up during the night.** Keep in mind that no matter what you do, there will be instances of getting up during the night, as the sleep cycle of the person with dementia changes.

STEP NINE: MAKE LIFE AS SIMPLE AS POSSIBLE

Consider other items. Would your loved one ring a bell for assistance? If so, place one on a nightstand next to the bed. Add a "ring for help" note if that would help.

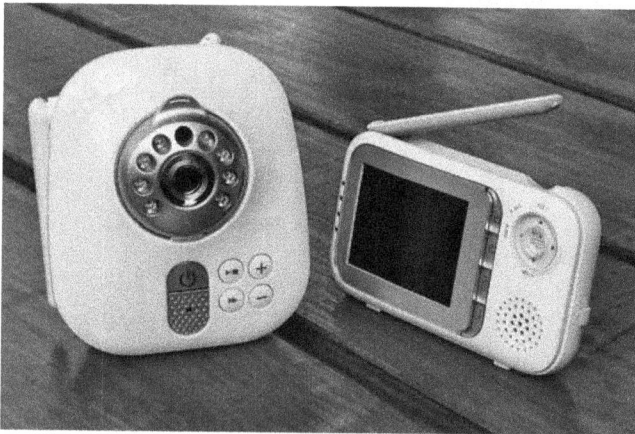

A simple baby monitor could do wonders for assuring safety.

Consider using a baby monitor to hear what might be happening in the room. Taking it further, an indoor surveillance system might be in order. If you do opt for a camera system, camouflage it in a plant or other item to detract attention from it. The progression of their dementia will help to determine what kind of monitoring devices, if any, you will need.

While putting all these safety measures in place, remember that the bedroom is your loved one's personal space.

- Decorate the room with favorite photos, books, and quilts.

- Make sure his or her favorite items are within view.
- Make sure their favorite magazines or books are accessible.
- Add decorations from the person's own home if he or she is moving in with you.
- Make the room as homey and familiar as possible to enhance a positive sense of wellbeing and belonging.

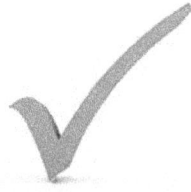

✓ CHAPTER TWO CHECKLIST

____ I have made the light switch easy to find and have removed bedside lamps.

____ I have eliminated poor wall colors, such as light blue, gray, or any dark colored paint.

____ I have removed trash cans from the bedroom.

____ I have installed an automatic light in the closet and reduced the number of clothing choices.

____ I have filled dresser drawers with personal items so that my loved one can rummage.

____ I am aware that my loved one may require a warmer room than the rest of the house.

____ I have looked into the possibility of a bed bar or pressure sensitive pad.

____ I have installed nightlights and a lit pathway for when my loved one needs to use the bathroom.

____ I have checked that all carpet is secure, reducing the risk of falls.

____ I have made their bedroom feel like home, keeping it as familiar and comfortable as possible.

CHAPTER THREE
THE BATHROOM

Although your loved one will not be hanging out in the bathroom, it's a room that is used often and poses some of the greatest risks in the house. Before your loved one uses this space, you need to address potential safety concerns.

Keep a comforting and homey environment in mind. Although you may need some fixtures or equipment that are used in institutions, try to avoid a hospital-like setting.

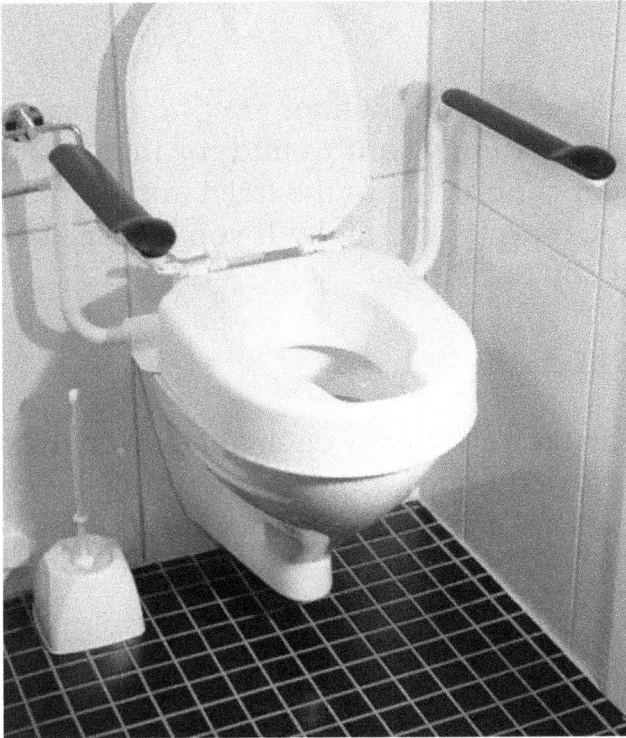

Any device assistance that helps getting on and off a toilet will benefit your loved one.

Remember, you want your loved one to feel comfortable and at ease.

STEP ONE: MAKE THE BATHROOM EASY TO LOCATE

First, it is necessary to make sure that the bathroom is easy to locate. This will help prevent frustration and possible accidents that have to be cleaned up when the bathroom cannot be found.

We've already mentioned putting a label on the bathroom door. Before that, though, there could be a walk to the bathroom, perhaps down a long hallway. Here are some basic tips:

- **The hallway should have enough light.** Nightlights ensure the individual can navigate his or her way to the bathroom after dark.

- **Installing handrails in the hallway will give your loved one stability.** Installing them on one side of the hall may be enough.

- **Hang signs on the walls with arrows pointing to the bathroom.** This may help the person find the bathroom. The bathroom door should be kept open at night while doors to other rooms should be closed to discourage wandering into them.

- **Look at the colors in the bathroom.** Is everything white? Having the same color throughout the bathroom will make things hard to find for the person with dementia. A floor with some color contrasting to the toilet and bathtub will be a great help in finding the toilet, especially at night. If you have a linoleum floor, it will be easier and less costly to change.

STEP TWO: MAKE IT EASY TO ENTER AND EXIT THE BATHROOM

Once your loved one gets to the bathroom, can they effectively enter and exit on their own? The bathroom door itself could be a barrier. Older people have trouble gripping, so knobs become a problem. Door levers are *much* easier to turn than knobs.

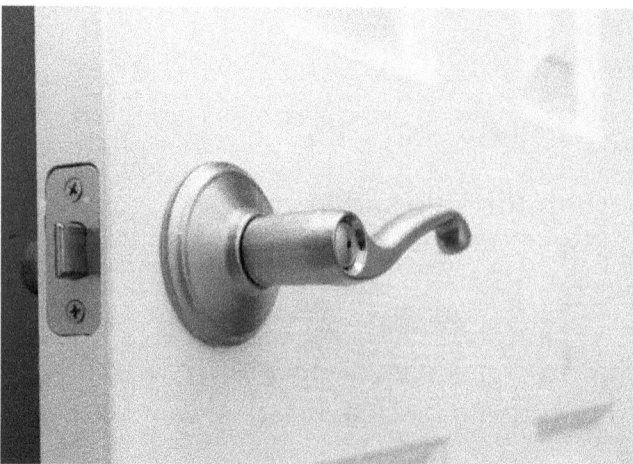

Lever door handles are easier to see and use.

If the door continues to be in the way, it may be necessary to remove it completely. If so, hang a curtain in the doorway that is easy to move aside. It may be something to get used to, even for the person with dementia, but this adjustment may be necessary to facilitate ease in entering and exiting the bathroom.

STEP THREE: PROVIDE ENOUGH LIGHTING

Just as lighting is important in the bedroom, a well-lit bathroom is equally important. Make sure there is plenty of lighting to help older eyes.

- **An easy-to-find light switch is a must.** Again, you can find glow-in-the-dark switch plates that will help.

- **Always have a night light or two, depending on the size of the room.** Having nightlights may be enough to keep the person from trying to find the light switch for the overhead light. Sometimes it may make sense to leave the bathroom light on all the time, making the bathroom easy to find.

- **Dim showers can even be lit up with specialty built-in lights.** This type of alteration will require an electrician.

STEP FOUR: MAKE THE FLOORING SAFE

Many tile floors are very slippery once they get wet. To see if this is the case, wet your floors and test them. If they are slippery, apply a non-skid material that will help. However, you may decide to go with another type of flooring completely.

- An alternative to bathroom tile or linoleum is removable, washable carpet. Having carpet lessens the possibility of slipping on wet tile while providing the room with a warmer look and feel. If you do opt for carpet, look for carpet with a surface that is easy to clean.

- Apply *Scotchgard* to a bathroom carpet or hire a professional to do it. This will help protect carpet from accidents and make cleaning easier. Some long-term care facilities use carpet that comes in squares for easy replacement should a section of the carpet become damaged.

Whatever you decide on the flooring, make sure the surface is smooth throughout the bathroom. Check the threshold into the bathroom to make sure it isn't a different height from the flooring. Finally, remove throw rugs if falling is a hazard. While throw rugs are a practical and warm bathroom accessory, they contribute to tripping and falling, which could result in injury on a hard bathroom floor.

STEP FIVE: MAKE ANY CHANGES TO THE TOILET, TUB, AND SHOWER

Finding the toilet is one of the most important considerations in the bathroom. Spend some time looking at your options, as a stress-free toileting experience will make a significant difference in the wellbeing of the person with Alzheimer's.

- **If the toilet is too low and hard for the individual to get up from, adjust the height with a toilet riser**. A bedside commode also works well for raising the toilet and providing something to hold onto. Grab bars can be installed in key places to aid with sitting down and getting back up.

- **Purchasing a colorful toilet seat or cover for the toilet lid will help distinguish the toilet from its surroundings.** This makes it much easier for the person to find.

- **Make the toilet comfortable.** You can replace a hard seat with a soft one. A cold, hard seat in the middle of the night might deter the person from using the bathroom, which could lead to an accident. You can also purchase "comfort height" toilets that sit higher and are easier to get on and off.

- **Consider a bidet.** The bidet is common in many countries, and a bidet attachment can be easily installed to your existing toilet. They provide a spray of water to the bottom area allowing for faster and easier clean up.

- **Install a grab bars.** This makes getting off and on the toilet easier and safer.

- **If there are glass doors, remove them and replace them with a shower curtain**. Again, grab bars are your friend. Install them in and around the shower and tub.

- **Have a shower seat available and install a shower hose**. If needed, individuals can shower while sitting down. This will also be highly beneficial when they require assistance bathing. A handheld showerhead will make cleaning "hard to reach" areas much easier when helping the confused or uncooperative person.

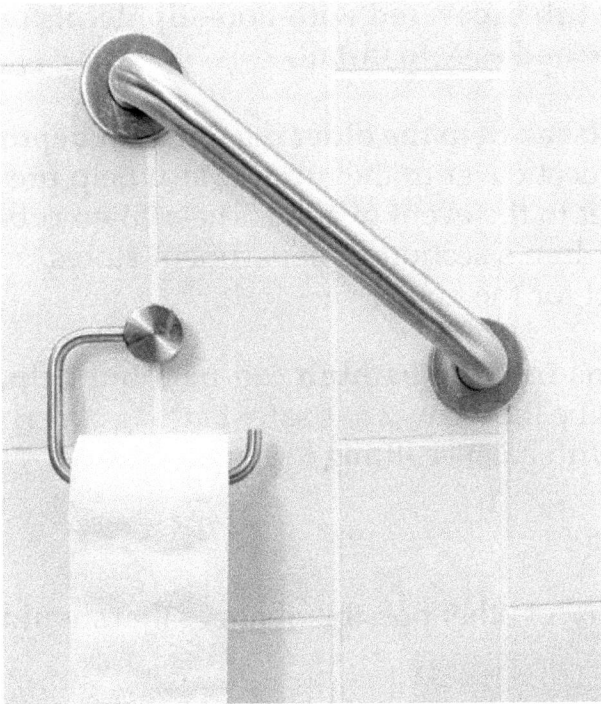

Grab bars are good for both beside a toilet and in a shower.

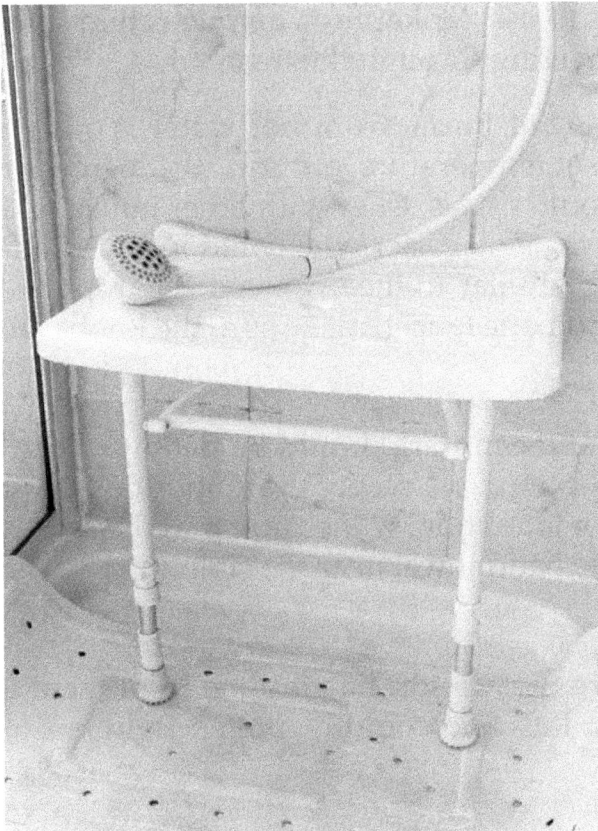

The ability to sit in a shower will make the showering process safer and less stressful.

- **Make sure the floor of the shower or tub is covered with non-slip decals or a non-skid mat**. These are inexpensive and easy to install.

- **A brightly colored floor mat in the tub can help the older person with depth perception.** Adding a foam rubber faucet cover in the tub will also help prevent injury if the person hits the faucet in the event of a fall. These foam rubber covers are often found in the children's section of department stores, as they are a general child-safety product for the home.

- **A walk-in tub with a door that opens into the bathtub can be a big help.** While these tubs are costly, they could be the answer to a safer bathing experience for the person who has trouble with balance lifting legs up.

STEP SIX: ADDRESS OTHER NECESSARY CHANGES

Each living environment differs, so here is a list of other possible changes that should be made.

- **Remove the trash can to prevent toileting in it**. It is unfortunate, but it happens. If this bathroom is shared with other family members, put the trash can in the cabinet under the sink for others to use. Make sure you put a child safety lock on the cabinet to prevent rummaging through the trash.

- **Install an anti-scalding device to prevent burns from hot water**. You can adjust your hot water heater to a pre-set temperature, around 105 degrees or so, but the lower water temperature could cause issues with other household needs. To make using the water from the sink easier, you could install a faucet that goes on and off automatically, similar to the ones you see in public restrooms. If you don't go with the automatic faucet, make sure the knobs are easy to turn and are within reach.

- **Sharp corners on bathroom cabinets and counters should be padded**. Foam pipe insulation is an easy, affordable option. Just secure it around the edges. A recessed counter, while a more major alteration, will ensure that the sink is reachable. Be sure to have an accessible hand towel near the sink, too.

- **Replace towel bars in locations where they might be grabbed to prevent a fall**. Flimsy towel racks won't prevent falls and could be pulled right out of the wall. Replace them with grab bars.

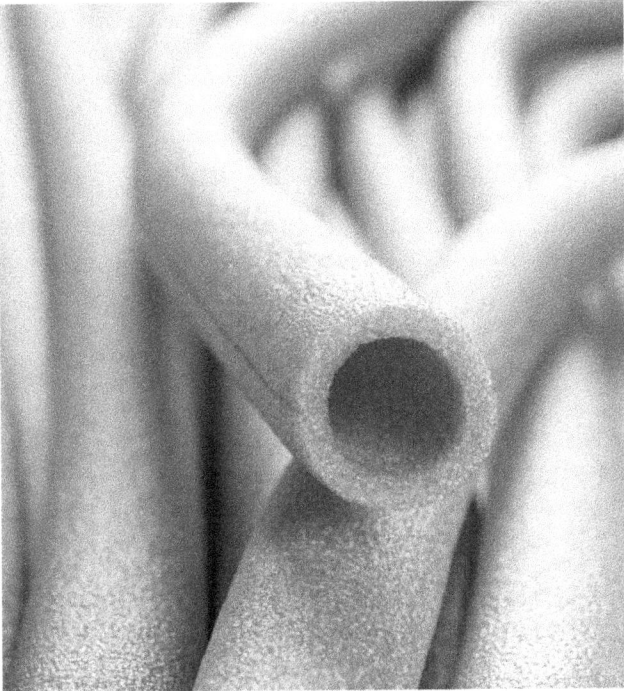

While it may look out of place, if your loved one is prone to falling, covering sharp edges and corners of vanities with low-cost foam pipe insulation might reduce the risk of injury.

- **Add a small drain screen to the sink.** This will save anything—such as valuable rings—from going down the drain.

- **If your loved one can still shave, provide him with an electric shaver away from the sink**. An old-fashioned razor is out of the question, but an electric shaver allows a level of independence that a man will appreciate. Make sure it is rechargeable and doesn't require an electrical cord next to the sink.

- **Cover or remove mirrors.** This is important if the individual's image confuses or frightens him or her. As dementia progresses, people think of themselves as younger than they are. They may not recognize themselves in the mirror. It is not uncommon to have a person leave a bathroom and say, "There's a stranger in there." Cover windows with blinds or curtains. Remove any breakable items from the counters. Remove any wall hooks, such as those for robes or towels that the person could fall into.

- **Place locks on medicine cabinets or remove unsafe items completely.** Everyday items you are accustomed to having in the bathroom now present a threat. This could include: mouthwash, nail polish, medications of any kind, perfumes, cleaning supplies, etc. Locks should go on any cabinets that contain chemicals, even personal items such as shampoo. One place a lock should not go, however, is on the door inside the bathroom. Don't risk your loved one getting locked in. If the bathroom has a window, add a safety lock there for additional security.

- **Install shelves for items that your loved one needs to access.** Shelves should be easily reached and sturdy (they may act as grab bars if your loved one were to slip). Such shelves could hold clean towels, facial tissues, and extra rolls of toilet paper. All family members should be instructed to keep any other items off those shelves to reduce confusion and a sense of feeling overwhelmed.

- **Remove glass items.** Ceramic items, glass shelving, drinking glasses — don't risk harm by having any of these in the bathroom. Replace glass shelves with wood, and glass cups with plastic.

- **Make the bathroom warm.** Never leave a person with dementia alone with a space heater; however, older people often feel colder than the average person, especially in the bathroom. Since many with dementia have aversions to bathing, the more you can do to make the bathroom comfortable, the better. Before the person takes a bath or shower, make sure the bathroom is warm — warmer than you would want it. If that involves bringing in a space heater, go ahead: just remove it before proceeding with the bath. Instead of a space heater, you could install heating lamps in the ceiling. This option, a job which may require an electrician, is much safer. If exhaust fans are already installed, make sure to keep them turned off when the person is in the bathroom. Excess noise can cause confusion, so keep the bathroom as calm and quiet as possible.

- **As the level of care provided for the person with Alzheimer's increases, a mechanical chair lift is an option that may be needed down the road.** Getting on and off the toilet will get harder, as will be getting in and out of the shower or tub. Lifts will aid in safety transferring the individual from a wheelchair to the toilet and back, as well as to the bathtub and back. While mechanical lifts are expensive and take up some room, they are a lifesaver and a back saver.

With more equipment in place, the bathroom has the tendency to become more institutional-looking. Paint and carpet, or other flooring options, should be warm colors which will help ward off this look. Maintain the homey look and feel as much as possible with personal touches like familiar pictures on the wall and pretty curtains on the windows. Even colorful, fluffy towels will help maintain the feel of home.

As care needs increase, you will need to take more measures to ensure that needs are met. These interventions will be easier to implement since you will already have a number of safety measures in place. In the beginning, start with the adjustments you can make to ensure the bathroom is as safe as it can possibly be without sacrificing a home-like environment. When you need to add more, you will know in advance what that will be—and you will be prepared.

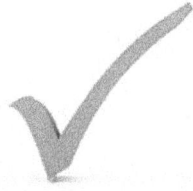

✔ CHAPTER THREE CHECKLIST

_____ I have ensured that there is enough light at nighttime in order to find the bathroom.

_____ I have made changes to the bathroom door so that it is no longer a barrier.

_____ I have removed or concealed trash cans.

_____ I have made the toilet comfortable and easy-to-use.

_____ I have installed grab bars within the shower.

_____ I have placed a colorful, non-slip mat in the tub.

_____ I have added a screen to the sink drain.

_____ I have placed a lock on the medicine cabinet and have removed all cleaning supplies.

_____ I have considered installing heat lamps in the ceiling to reduce reliance on a space heater.

CHAPTER FOUR
THE LIVING AREA

The living areas, such as living rooms and dens, should be safe and comfortable gathering places for families. The person with dementia needs to feel part of the family and the rooms must accommodate his or her needs.

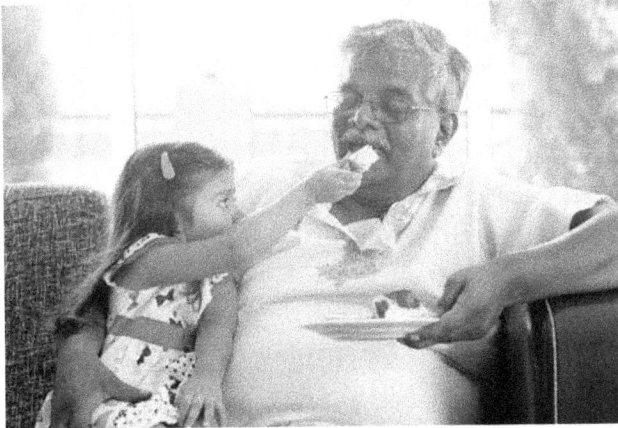

Having a safe and comfortable environment that minimizes chances of frustration and injury will help your family member feel at ease.

STEP ONE: FOCUS ON THE SPACE ITSELF

Make sure the living area has plenty of space to roam with clear pathways. This may require getting rid of some of the furniture, such as extra chairs, side tables, and bookcases. First, look for the furniture that might be removed for its danger factor.

- **Moreover, remove anything that obstructs a clear path.** This includes foot stools and furniture.

- **Reduce clutter.** Too much clutter can cause confusion and agitation. Remove as much clutter as possible to make the space roomier. Trash cans, statues, and floor lamps can be in the way and serve as trip hazards. Stacks of magazines and newspapers can be overwhelming. Put DVDs and CDs in enclosed cabinets or drawers in tables, or store them in another room. Put remotes in a drawer.

STEP TWO: LOOK AT YOUR FURNITURE

Look at the furniture for usability and safety.

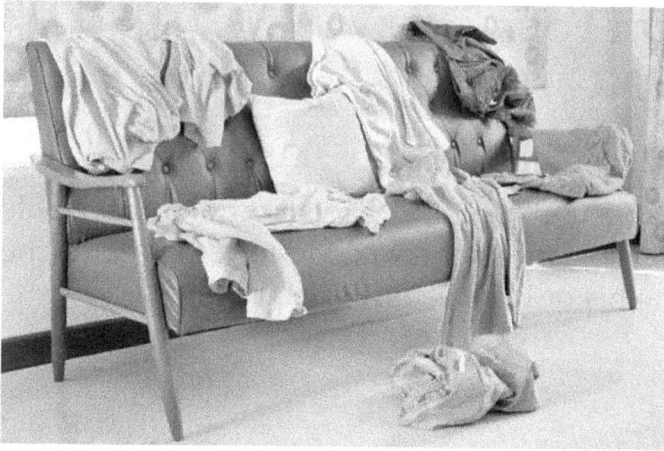

Clutter around the house makes for tripping hazards and a feeling of greater disorganization.

- **Address sharp edges.** Is there furniture with sharp edges that could pose a danger? If so, can you live without them in order to make the room more spacious and safe? If not, consider padding the edges. There are low-cost products to help with this.

- **Get rid of wobbly furniture.** If your loved one leans on the furniture, it needs to support him or her. Furniture with glass that could be easily broken should be removed.

- **Seating should be firm and sturdy.** Do chairs have arms for the older person to hold onto when getting up? If the seat needs to be higher, consider adding a firm cushion to the chair for added height.

- **Protect upholstery from spills.** Use a heavy-duty substance, such as *Scotchgard*. Alternatively, use slipcovers to protect expensive furniture.

- **Rolling chairs should be removed.** Consider removing rocking chairs, too. They are not the best choice for a person with balance issues. Still, a rocking chair is something older people often use in their own homes, and the rocking action is generally soothing. Some rocking chairs are safer than others, so you don't have to rule them out.

- **Look into getting a lift chair if needed.** Your loved one may be used to relaxing in a recliner. If this is the case, but getting up from one is a problem, the lift chair may be your answer. You can buy a regular chair and order the lifting apparatus to attach to it. Check with the doctor for a recommendation. Medicare may pay for the attachable lifting mechanism.

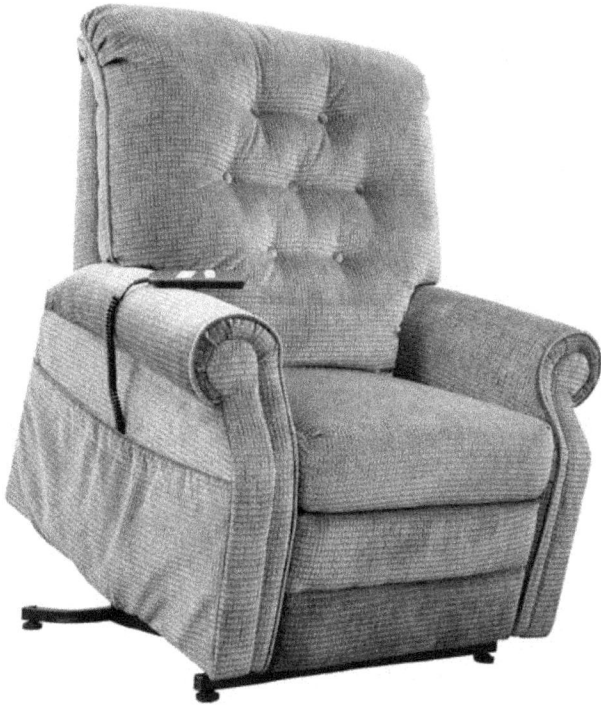

Like a hospital bed, as mobility decreases, a mechanical chair will help the individual feel independent and can save the caregiver's back from lifting.

- **Check tables for sturdiness**. Do end tables serve a purpose? Are they steady to the touch? Would they hold up if someone held onto them to prevent falling? If the answer to these questions is no, then you might need to remove them from the room.

- **Footstools and coffee tables pose a potential tripping hazard.** In addition, the person with dementia, not realizing how low the stools are to the ground, might sit on one and fall off or not be able to get back up. A contrasting color to the carpet will reduce the threat as a tripping hazard. Depending on the material of the table or stool, you could paint it to better contrast with the color of the carpet in order for the table to be easily spotted.

STEP THREE: FOCUS ON DECORATIONS

Decorations need to be addressed both in terms of safety and for comfort. You should remove any items that pose a threat, yet leave items that make your loved one feel at home.

- **Keep favorite items to make the room familiar and homey**. Things that are familiar might be a clock or a particular painting. Does he or she have favorite knick-knacks or collections?

- **Locking breakable items in a display case is an option.** If it gets to the point where seeing a prized collection but not being able to get to it becomes distressing, then it might be time to store the items out of sight. For the person with dementia, out of sight may be out of mind.

- **Look for heavy decorations that might be positioned throughout the room.** Bookends? Free-standing clocks? What about heavy books with prominent edges? Any of these items could become dangerous if the person with dementia were to become agitated and throw one in a fit of anger. Evaluate every item in the living room and throughout the house.

- **Never light candles in a home where someone with dementia roams.** If you enjoy the inviting warmth of candles, there are battery-powered candles that mimic the mood of real candles.

- **Remove any plants that could be toxic if eaten**. Check a list of plants that fall in this category, either online or by calling the Poison Control Center. Also, remove any small stones in the base of the pot, as they could be picked up and put in the mouth.

- **Remove any items with openings as such that could be perceived as a toilet**. Just as in the bathroom, or in any room, certain objects can be mistaken for a toilet. Flower pots are one of those items, as are magazine holders and umbrella stands.

STEP FOUR: ASSESS LIGHTING AND FANS

As in any room, the living room should be well-lit with bright bulbs overhead. If you must use table lamps, make sure the cords are out of the way. Long cords or extension cords can be tacked to the baseboards to keep them from being a trip hazard.

- **In lamps, replace incandescent bulbs with fluorescent.** Fluorescent bulbs won't get as hot to the touch should wandering hands land on them.

- **Lighting is affected by ceiling fans.** Check to see if the fan makes the light "jump" and throw shadows. Either can be distracting and irritating to a person with dementia.

- **Check ceiling fans for other factors.** Are they too low or too loose? Are they too loud? Loud noise is yet another assault on the senses that causes irritation. Even the draft from a fan, or "wind" perceived by the person with dementia, may be unsettling and uncomfortable to someone with altered perception.

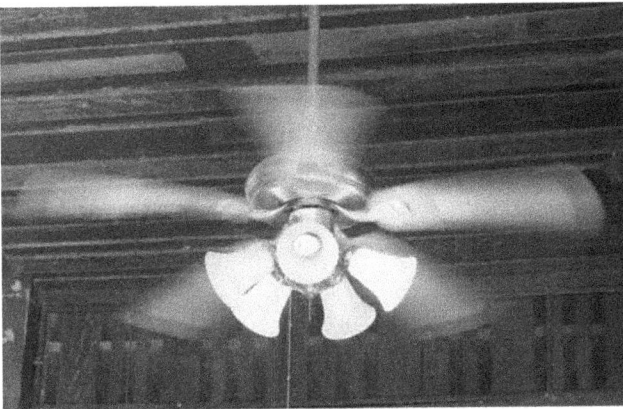

Loud and possibly casting shadows, ceiling fans should be used only if they don't contribute to confusion.

- **Close blinds and curtains at dark.** As daylight fades, windows and sliding glass doors will operate as mirrors by bouncing back the reflection of the on-looker.

STEP FIVE: DON'T FORGET POTENTIAL EXITS

Speaking of sliding glass doors, during the day, these glass doors may invite a person to wander out into the yard or garden. You must ensure that your loved one does not wander outside alone.

- **Make sure sliding glass doors or other exits are locked.** Locks can be installed up high or down low or both, making opening those more of a challenge. There are also low-cost door alarms that can be installed to notify you if they are opened.

- **Camouflaged exits keep the wanderer from recognizing the door as an exit.** In some dementia units within long-term care facilities, they hire an artist to paint a scene on exit doors that blends the door with the rest of the room, completely masking the appearance of an exit. This type of alteration may be too drastic for the look of your home, and it may cost more than what you are willing or able to pay. This practice, however, has been known to work in nursing homes. A lower-cost option may be painting the door the same color as the wall.

- **Door knob covers also prevent egress.** These low-cost covers can be found in the baby section of most department stores. They make turning the knob more of a challenge.

STEP SIX: ADDITIONAL TIPS

Depending on the needs of your loved one and the space in which you reside, you may need to implement some or all of the following suggestions. Use these to guide you through necessary changes.

- **Look at drapes or curtains.** While curtains definitely make a room appear homier, those with busy prints can be irritating to the person with Alzheimer's. Opt for solid colors for your curtains throughout the house.

- **If curtains are too long and could be tripped over, they should be shortened.** You might pull the curtains themselves back, while letting the blinds do the job of covering the windows after the sun goes down.

- **Purchase cord-safe products to shorten cords on blinds.** It seems there are potential dangers everywhere you turn, as the blinds present yet another hazard with the cord that hangs down. Avoid the temptation for anyone to want to play with the cord, or, worse, to get wrapped up in it. These provide an out-of-the-way place to wrap cords and keep them from dangling.

- **Make sure carpeting is secure and smooth.** An individual with dementia scoots his or her feet and can thus stumble over ripples in the carpet. Likewise, area rugs, since they are not flush with the floor, can present a tripping hazard. Have you ever seen area rugs in a nursing home resident's room? There is a reason for that.

- **Hardwood floors can be dangerous if they are not level.** This may be a problem in older homes. Remember that hardwood floors should not be too shiny or easily slid on.

- **Prevent accidents before they happen.** Look around to see what could be a danger. Cover the fireplace with a protective guard. Attach padding to the edges. Are you afraid of your flat-screen TV getting knocked over? Secure it with safety straps. If you are afraid of your loved trying to climb a bookcase or tipping over another heavy piece of furniture, tie it down.

- **Control the noise.** A lot of people keep the television on for much of the day. Noise is an irritant to someone with dementia and can encourage agitation or aggression, thus spurring on efforts to leave the area. Instead of playing the TV, try soothing music for your loved one. Don't leave anything—even music—playing all the time, though, as constant stimulation can bring on agitation as well. Similarly, if you have a home telephone, turn down the ringer volume to minimize confusion and keep the person with Alzheimer's from trying to answer the phone.

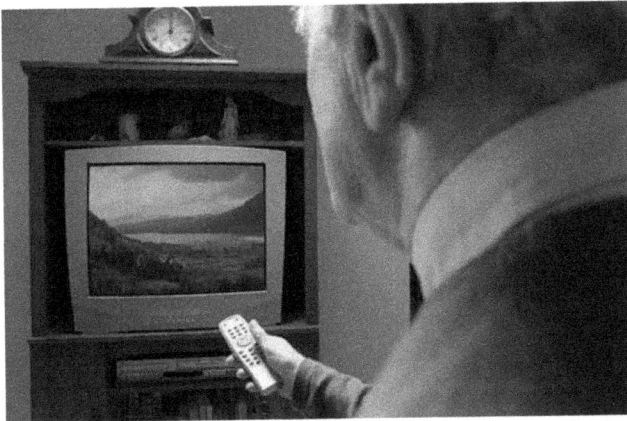

Beyond background noise, television shows may cause confusion. Is that war movie the news? Who is that person talking to me?

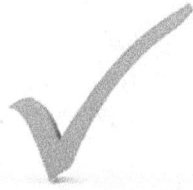

✔ CHAPTER FOUR CHECKLIST

____ I removed all wobbly furniture and furniture with glass.

____ I checked all furniture for sturdiness.

____ I eliminated anything that could cause trips or falls.

____ Breakable items are put away, locked up, or are kept in place using an adhesive.

____ Heavy or sharp items have been removed and put away in a safe location.

____ Long cords have been tacked to baseboards and toxic plants have been removed.

____The living room is well-lit and ceiling fans are safe and quiet.

____Anything that could be mistaken as a toilet has been removed.

CHAPTER FIVE
THE KITCHEN

Along with the bathroom, the kitchen is one of the most dangerous rooms in the house for someone with dementia. Sharp knives, breakable dishes, small and large appliances, and hot surfaces present dangers.

In most homes, the kitchen is also a popular gathering place, a warm and inviting room where families and guests spend a lot of quality time together, connecting through food and conversation. It is imperative to pay special attention to making the kitchen as safe as possible to include your loved one's use of the space.

STEP ONE: SURVEY THE LOOK AND FUNCTIONALITY OF THE KITCHEN

As with the other rooms, survey the kitchen's general look and feel. Look at the big picture as you assess the room. Peruse the space to make sure pathways are clear for someone wandering in and out. Kitchens are often a high-traffic room for families so it's important for this space to be functional, yet safe.

- **Make sure chairs are easy to get in and out of and within earshot of kitchen happenings.** If the kitchen is generally where a lot of family time is spent, try to include a chair for your loved one to sit near the action, where he or she will feel a part of things. Also, make sure there is enough padding. If the chair is too hard on their bottom, this could cause this area to fall asleep, which would make walking even more challenging.

- **Good lighting in the kitchen, as in other rooms, is necessary to aid in daily activities.** We all need to see what we are eating at mealtimes, but this is ever more important for the person with dementia. Vision and perception in the older person may be continually changing, which can be further impacted by dim lighting. Make sure lighting is adequate overhead and that night lighting includes a night light or two, depending on the size of the kitchen.

- **Look at kitchen flooring with a critical eye.** Kitchen floors get wet, particu-larly in front of the sink, so consider this when assessing safety. If your floors are tile, you may have to apply or hire someone to apply a non-skid adhesive on top. For linoleum or hardwood, assess for safety by wetting the floor. Apply some type of covering if it is slippery when wet.

- **Make sure kitchen furniture is comfortable and sturdy.** Dining chairs should have arms to assist getting in and out of them. The dining table should be sturdy to the touch. Pedestal tables are dangerous if someone tries to climb on top of them. Consider removing them.

- **Cover the table with a tablecloth that contrasts with the floor if it is shiny.** The shine can be irritating and bothersome.

- **Other furniture besides the dining table can pose a threat.** You might consider removing furnishings such as baker's racks and footstools, both of which can be used for climbing. Plain bar stools might be in the way while also being a seating hazard. Without arms, it is much easier for the older person to slip off onto the floor.

STEP TWO: MAKE SURE APPLIANCES DO NOT THREATEN SAFETY

- **The stove is one of the biggest dangers in the kitchen.** Remove the knobs when the stove is not in use or install a switch to turn off the power. Cover the burners when not in use to detract attention.

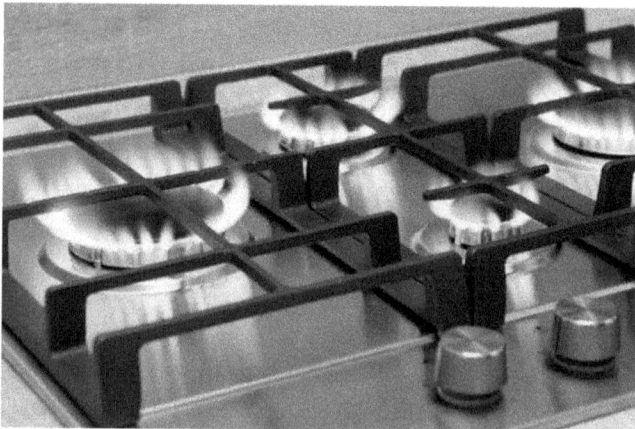

Any open flame is a danger, and many people are accustomed to cooking out of habit. Be careful.

- **The oven is a major concern.** Putting a lock on it may be the best way to ensure the individual's safety and the caregiver's peace of mind. Appliance locks are easily attached and automatically lock when set to the "on" position. Lock it when off, too. You might be surprised how many older people stop using their ovens for cooking but use them for storing kitchen items, such as pots and pans. This might work just fine until the oven goes on and melts pot handles and whatever else might be inside.

- **Limit access to the microwave.** The person with dementia does not realize that putting metal or aluminum in a microwave can start a fire. He or she may put items in and turn on the timer for hours, resulting in burned food or objects and a potential fire hazard.

- **The refrigerator may pose a danger.** Place items your loved one might need on a shelf that is easy to reach and at eye level. If the dementia has progressed to the point where free access to the refrigerator is dangerous, it may be necessary to lock it up along with the stove. The person with dementia might eat raw food, old food, or drop breakable jars.

- **Small appliances can pose a danger, too.** Unplug them and insert safety plugs into the outlets. If you have room in the cabinets, consider removing appliances (when reasonable) from the counters and placing them there. Look into small appliances that shut off automatically. You can get coffeemakers and tea kettles, for instance, which shut off automatically. Keep small appliances away from the sink to avoid any contact with water.

STEP THREE: ADDRESS THE SINK AND GARBAGE DISPOSAL

- **This garbage disposal is a definite danger if kept connected.** Disconnecting it will ensure that items aren't stuffed down the sink or, worse, that human hands get mangled. If you don't want to stop using the disposal, spend the money to buy one with a safety feature. There are garbage disposals on the market that will not run unless a cover is in place. This invention works differently than the traditional disposal which requires water running down the drain while grinding. With the way this one works, fingers, silverware, or other small items cannot get chopped up. This is a wonderful appliance for households with children or cognitively impaired individuals. Another plus—this apparatus is also quiet.

- **Automatic faucets and anti-scalding devices also work well in the kitchen.** If you do not have an automatic shut-off device on your faucet, hide the sink stoppers to prevent the sinks from getting clogged and overflowing.

- **Add drain screens to prevent losing anything down the drain.**

STEP FOUR: FOCUS ON CABINETS AND CUPBOARDS

A number of potential dangers are lurking in your kitchen cabinets. There are dishes that can be broken, heavy pots that can fall on a toe, and food, including spices, that shouldn't be eaten without being cooked. Dangers linger with sharp knives, cleaning supplies, and plastic bags. Yes, plastic bags. A seemingly innocuous plastic trash bag can become a choking or suffocation hazard in seconds.

- **The easiest way to prohibit access to these types of items is to install child-proof safety latches on all the cabinets.** These are inexpensive and easy to install.

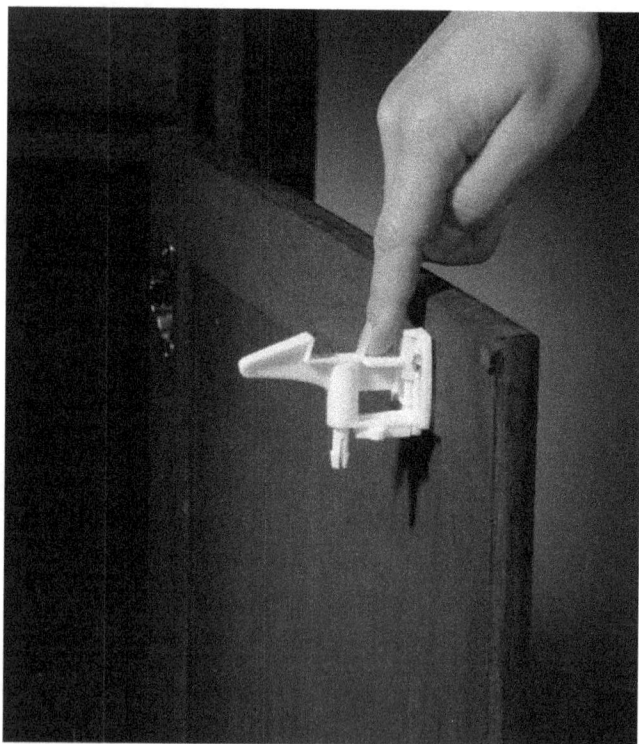

Household cleaners under the kitchen sink? A simple child safety latch will help ensure safety.

- **Cabinets may also be camouflaged by painting the cabinet pulls a color similar to that of the cabinets.** Be mindful that denying access to kitchen cabinets could cause frustration to the person with Alzheimer's making his or her way to the kitchen for a snack. If your loved one is capable of going to the kitchen and making a snack, creating a safe environment to allow this will afford your loved one greater independence. Consider loading a few shelves or drawers with certain foods. Stock designated locations with snack items such as crackers, cookies, granola bars, fruit, or any other favorites.

- **Label cabinets with words such as "snacks" or a picture of foods if the ability to read has declined.** Lettering should be large and bold with a block font as opposed to script.

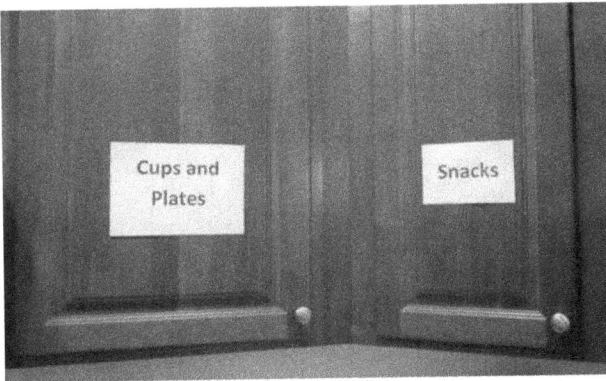

Kitchen cabinets can blend together to the person with Alzheimer's. Labeling the cabinets' contents will help navigating where to go for what.

STEP FIVE: EATING AND DINING

There are hazards in the kitchen that you may not realize. A person with Alzheimer's will often get to the point where they will eat a number of non-edible items.

- **Do you have a bowl of artificial fruit?** Remove it. In fact, you might remove a bowl of real fruit if eating too much of it becomes a problem.

- **Refrigerator magnets can also pose a danger.** Small magnets that look like food might be mistaken for just that, and swallowed.

- **Check your counters and windowsills for other small items that could be swallowed.** Remove them from the kitchen.

- **Look at colors.** Distinguishing food from the plate that holds it may become more difficult. Colored plates may help highlight the food for your loved one.

- **There are a number of adaptive items you can purchase to make your loved**

one's dining experience easier and more pleasant. As people get older, their diminished motor skills makes forks and drinking glasses harder to hold and manipulate. With dementia, cognitive issues affect perception and understanding, as well. The person may be confused about how to use the objects in front of him or her, or embarrassed that he/she cannot hold his/her spoon steady.

- **Keep all alcohol in a locked cabinet.** Drinking alcohol can increase confusion.

You've looked at the lighting and the dining area itself. Now, look further into the details that go into creating an ideal eating experience.

As with any other room, color contrast is helpful. You've made sure the table does not blend in with the floor, perhaps with the aid of a tablecloth. If you use placemats, make sure that the color contrasts with the tablecloth and with the plates. People with dementia have a hard time perceiving boundaries when colors blend together. Being able to find their food will make eating easier. Here are a few more tips:

- **Purchase non-skid placemats and non-skid dishes.** This is just an extra safety measure to prevent accidents. Specialty plates include those with high rims or bumper guards to keep food from being pushed over the edges onto the table.

- **A glass or mug is never a good idea unless it is heavy-duty and non-breakable.** It may be hard to figure out just the right size of cup that is easy for the older, arthritic hand to hold. Consider investing in specialty cups that are ergonomically shaped for easier gripping. Some come with built-in straws that make drinking easier.

- **Adaptive utensils also come in many different forms.** Weighted forks and spoons are common in nursing homes, as they help steady the fork. All these items not only ensure safer dining, but they also afford the people with dementia as much independence as they can handle for as long as they are able.

- **Remove heavy pots and pans if you're loved one is still cooking or helping you in the kitchen.** Heavy-duty ceramic pots, for instance, are extremely heavy. If your loved one tries to picks these up, they could become injured.

After all of this, if you're still worried about your loved one getting into trouble in the kitchen, you can install a motion detector that will alarm when he or she goes into the room.

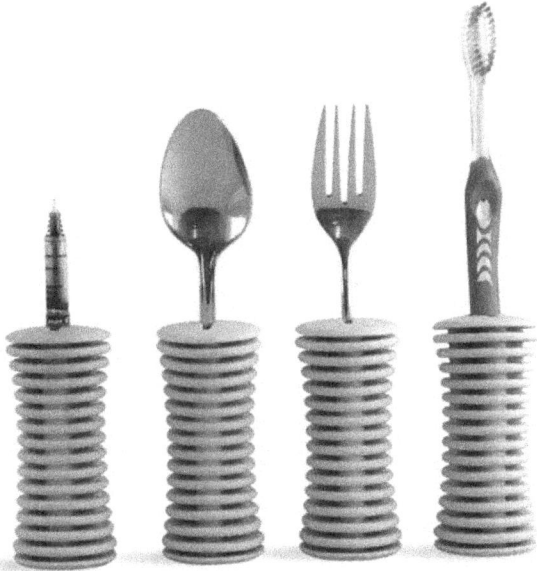

Large-handle utensils don't cost much and they can be very helpful.

If you do buy an in-home camera surveillance system, definitely include the kitchen in your monitoring. The noise from a motion detector can be an annoyance, so the best monitor for causing the least amount of distress may be a simple, low-cost baby monitor. Just have a monitor with you where you can hear if something inappropriate is going on in the kitchen.

Finally, have a fire extinguisher handy. Something unexpected can happen despite your best efforts. Make sure a smoke and fire detector is installed with fresh batteries that are frequently checked.

Having the ability to take care of one's self will maintain the highest level of functioning in your loved one for a while longer. Allowing access to familiar items will afford the person some freedom and sense of being in control of his or her own life, which will make them happier.

As your loved one's illness progresses, however, there may come a time when the kitchen is just too dangerous and must be added to the list of rooms that are off-limits, at least without supervision.

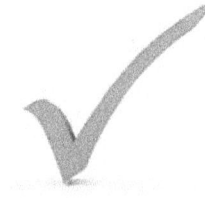

✓ CHAPTER FIVE CHECKLIST

_____ I have assessed the kitchen floors and ensured that tile is no longer slippery.

_____ I have checked all furniture to see that it is sturdy, including tables and dining chairs.

_____ I have made my oven, stove, and microwave safe by locking these appliances.

_____ I have reduced dangers associated with the garbage disposal and sink, including water temperature.

_____ I have labeled drawers to make items and food more accessible.

_____ Long cords have been tacked to baseboards and toxic plants have been removed.

_____ I have read about the challenges that can be encountered when eating and have made necessary changes.

_____ I have locked all alcohol up.

_____ I have a fire extinguisher ready.

_____ I have installed a home monitor which covers the kitchen area.

CHAPTER SIX
HALLWAYS AND ENTRYWAYS

If your home has a long hallway, you may have to make some adjustments to provide a safe and easy passage for someone with dementia. If there is no bathroom in your loved one's bedroom, the hallway will be especially important in leading him or her from his bed to the bathroom, a walk that becomes increasingly difficult as the sun goes down. Here are a few tips and suggestions:

- **Plug in a night light, or even two.** Hallways can be dark even during daylight hours. As in all the other rooms, make sure the lighting is bright enough to see one's way. Install sufficient overhead lighting if necessary, as well as nightlights that come on any time the light is too dim to see well.

- **As with other rooms, check the flooring.** Whether carpet or hardwood, make sure it is even and won't be tripped on.

- **Installing handrails, at least on one side of the hallway, may help an elderly person more easily navigate a long hallway.** As previously mentioned, this is especially important to lead the person from the bedroom to the bathroom.

- **Bedroom doors may be better off closed so they don't draw attention, day and night.** Try labeling, whether with words or with pictures, the doors to the rooms that your loved one will go to most often.

- **Many older homes have the water heater in a hall closet.** If this is the case in your house, put a lock on the door to prohibit access.

- **Check for floor vents or registers in which a walker or cane could get stuck.** Check your entire house to see if there are any other floor vents that are right in the walkway, covering them as needed.

- **Check the width of the doorways.** Are the doorways to key rooms wide enough? Will a wheelchair or walker fit through? Hopefully, you won't have to make any major alterations, but if the doors to the bathroom and other necessary rooms do not allow easy access, you may have to hire someone to widen the entryways.

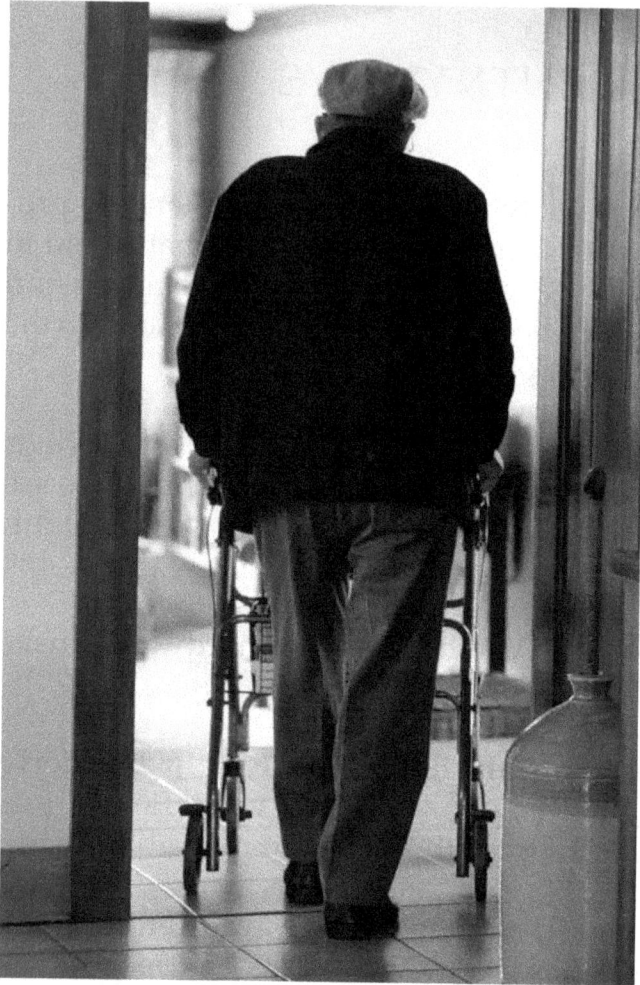

Widening doorways may not be cheap or easy, but if your house allows for it and walkers or wheelchairs are needed, it may be an important change to make.

- **While you're checking the doorways, also check the thresholds to make sure they are level to the floor.** Check the entrance to each room. Smooth down or replace thresholds with higher or lower ones as needed to make the flooring flush on both sides of the door. If there is a height difference, the threshold could present a tripping hazard.

- **If the hallway is narrow and has pictures on the wall, or if pictures hang close to the handrail, consider moving them and any decorations that can be bumped and knocked off.** You might be able to raise pictures that could be fallen into, as well as any decorations that might cause harm.

- **If the hallway is wide and long, place a chair or bench halfway for resting.**

Most hallways probably will not accommodate a chair, however. In that case, is there room for one immediately at the end of the hall? Depending on your home's layout, you may or may not be able to put a chair at each end of the hallway.

- **Entryways must also be considered.** They must be free of clutter. Remove items that might be in the way, such as decorative items, umbrella stands, and errant shoes that may have been left by family members. If there is room, placing a chair would be beneficial to provide a resting place for the elderly person who has just come in the door.

The hallways and entryways may seem like insignificant areas to consider in safe-proofing a house for the person with Alzheimer's. They are very important areas, however, as they lead to all the other rooms of the house. The hallway will play an important role in how your loved one navigates from the bedroom through-out the rest of the house. Similarly, the entryway is the first part of the house that is seen, inviting the person to a safe, secure home.

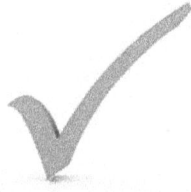

✔ CHAPTER SIX CHECKLIST

_____ I have placed nightlights in areas where light is dim.

_____ I have installed handrails in the hallway.

_____ I have placed arrows or labels throughout the hallway for navigation purposes.

_____ I have checked entryways and doorways, ensuring they're wide enough.

_____ I have removed pictures from the walls that may be knocked off and broken.

_____ I have assessed my loved one's needs in terms of my hallways, adding a chair if necessary.

_____ I have removed clutter from the entryways, including umbrella stands, shoes, and decorations.

_____ I have placed a chair at the main entryway so my loved one can rest when he or she gets in the door.

CHAPTER SEVEN

THE EXTERIOR

Once you've safety-proofed the inside of the house, don't forget the exterior. Peruse the whole yard, all the surroundings of your home, starting with the entrance. Walk the entire property through the eyes of someone looking for something to get into, something forbidden, or something that may cause harm.

Being able to go outside to enjoy the sights, sounds, and fresh air is a plus and health benefit to anyone, physically and emotionally. The same is true for the person with dementia. An outdoor area will provide a place to exercise, enjoy nature, and rest. Perhaps the outdoors is a non-issue, if you live in an apartment with no accessible outdoor areas. You can skip this chapter if that's the case. If not, read on.

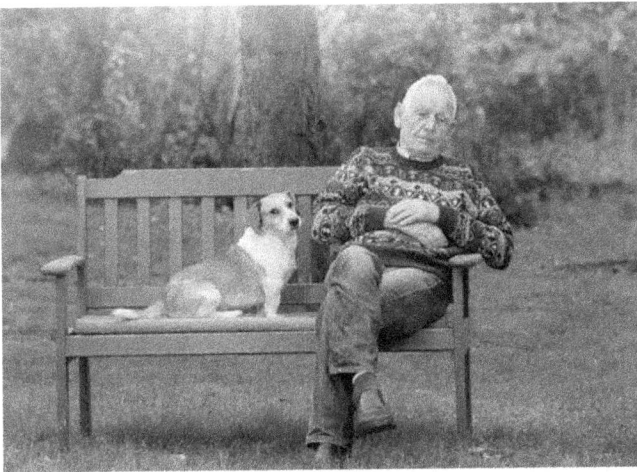

Sitting outside listening to sounds and watching birds is a pleasant way to pass time.

If your yard is not enclosed by a fence, then it may have to be off-limits. In that case, it will be necessary to keep exterior doors locked at all times, with locks out of reach to the person with dementia, very high or low where they may not be accustomed to looking for them.

On the other hand, if your loved one is going to have access to the outdoors, you will have your work cut out for you to ensure that the yard is free from potential hazards. Having a fenced area is only the beginning. Here are some suggestions and further information to ensure optimal safety.

START WITH THE ENTRYWAY

Making the outdoors safe for the person with dementia can be a challenge. It is harder to provide smooth walkways outdoors than it is to do inside the house. If you want your loved one to have access to the outdoors, however, it will be necessary to make some changes in your yard.

Before looking at the area, which will likely be the backyard, start first with the entrance to the house. Viewing the front door, make sure the pathway that leads to it is clean and smooth.

- **Preferably, a walkway will lead up to the front door**.

- **If you have stepping stones, fill the spaces between them.** Make sure someone with an unsteady gait won't trip over uneven rocks.

- **Imagine navigating a walker to the door.** A bumpy rock path or an uneven lawn will be difficult for any older person, whether there is assistance available from another person or not. A trip leading to a subsequent fall is something you definitely want to avoid.

- **Make sure lighting illuminates the pathway all the way to the door.** A well-lit path will be helpful in ensuring a stress-free walk and safe arrival to the front door. Besides being a visual aid, the light will put off an inviting aura from the home. The person with Alzheimer's is often fearful of many things, dim lighting and darkness being paramount. Warm lighting that allows one to see his or her surroundings is one step toward alleviating any fears.

- **Creating a smooth pathway that circles around the enclosed part of the yard will provide a safe walking area and distract from other areas of the yard that might be more difficult to navigate.** A walking path should be circular with no forks in the path to cause confusing choices. Any pathway should also not have a dead end where the person has to make yet another decision about what to do. If the path does dead end because of a pre-existing sidewalk or other condition, provide an attractive area at the end with comfortable seating for a rest area.

How Safe Are the Steps and Porch Leading to the Entrance?

- **Steps to the door should be level and clear.** If steps are too narrow for the whole foot to be placed, consider tearing out the steps and replacing them with foot-wide steps that are easier for feet to land on, or a ramp to walk up.

- **A simple alteration that will help make the steps stand out better requires only a bit of paint.** One option is to paint the rise on the step a different color from the step itself. To make this job simpler, you could just paint the edges of the steps or mark them by lining them with reflective tape.

- **Handrails on the steps will also help ensure a safe arrival to the front door**. Make sure they are steady and can hold someone's full weight. If your loved one is in a wheelchair, you will have to completely replace the steps with a ramp to provide access to the house. A slip-resistant strip could add a touch of safety while also providing contrasting color.

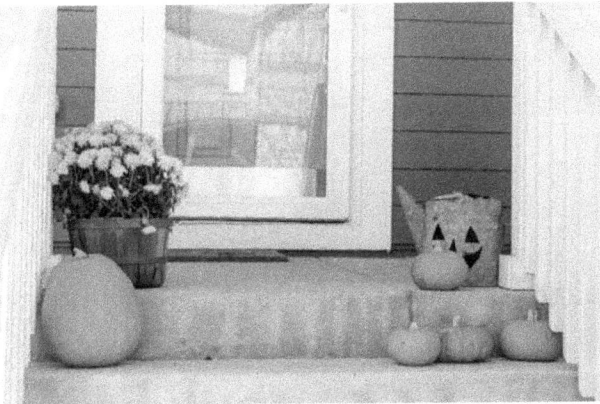

Beware of decorative items around stairs and walkways that could pose tripping hazards.

- **Have a chair on the front porch, if the space allows.** After a long walk to get to the front door, your loved one may be tired. If your pathway to the front is long, you might consider placing a bench along that walkway for a rest period halfway through. Having a chair just inside the home in an entryway could be a welcome respite as well. If space doesn't allow for this, get your loved one to the closest chair once you get him or her safely inside.

- **If your loved one is safe to be outdoors alone, he or she may still need help recognizing how to get back into the house.** Wandering around the pathway, unable to find the door back to the house, can cause confusion and fear in the person with dementia. Continuing to walk and search with a lack of awareness of being tired can also lead to injury as the result of a fall.

- **Put something recognizable next to the door that leads back into the house.** Something that is bright and inviting by the sliding glass doors or whatever other entrance will provide a landmark that can be spotted. Consider a bright chair or pot of flowers, a statue, or perhaps a charming birdhouse or chimes. Whatever you use, make sure it is easily seen from the walking path.

REMOVE ANYTHING THAT COULD CAUSE TRIPS OR FALLS

So many items present trip hazards in the yard—things you probably don't even think of. Look for rocks that stick up, whether big or small and remove them.

- **Roll up water hoses to keep them out of the way.**

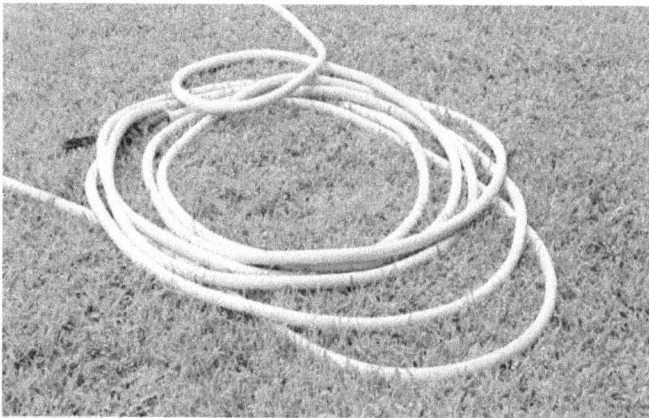

Like inside the house, reduce clutter outside the house.

- **Statues and figurines may pose trip hazards.** Move them and similar items to out-of-the-way places.

- **Make sure tools are picked up and locked away in the shed or garage.**

- **Potted plants are tripping hazards and present other hazards.** You will have to spend some time on the outside to research what plants might be toxic if eaten. Again, you can check the list the Poison Control Center puts out.

- **Trim plants that stick out and may trip or hit someone in the face.** Do this with all bushes and trees, trimming back to prevent poking and scratching.

EXAMINE GATES AND FENCING

A safe yard includes appropriate fencing that is sturdy and high. Check wood fences for rough surfaces that might have splinters. Sand any rough spots to protect bare hands. For metal fences, check for sharp edges and cover them. Whatever type of fence, it must be secure and able to withstand a person's weight against it.

Is the fence high enough? Six feet should be adequate. Shorter fences are just too tempting, as one can see over it into the neighbor's yard or the adjoining woods. To further ensure non-egress by way of the fence, chairs should not be placed close to the fence where they can be used for climbing to see what is on the other side.

Gates to the yard should be locked at all times. An alarm can be added for additional safety. Motion detectors can be installed in various areas to alert movement to certain areas of the yard. If the exit from your house is left unlocked for easy access to the backyard, add a bell or chimes to the door to signal that your loved one is going outside. Gates can be camouflaged by painting the latch the same color as the wood or perhaps hanging something that falls down over the latch.

AVOIDING POTENTIAL SERIOUS ACCIDENTS

There are a number of other dangers that lurk in the yard.

- **Swimming pools should be emptied and covered when not in use.** Still, anyone can fall onto a covered pool and have trouble getting back up, particularly the more confused and frail older adult. If a fence is not already surrounding the swimming pool, it may have to be installed, particularly if your loved one is allowed to roam in the yard unsupervised.

- **People have been known to drown in only a few inches of water, so consider this even if your pool is merely a small decorative one with goldfish.** Instead of getting rid of it, you might be able to keep your loved one out of harm's way by putting decorative fencing around this type of area.

- **Look around for other potential dangers in your backyard.** What about your backyard grill? Covering up barbecue grills might be enough to keep attention from them. Gas grills, however, offer another temptation with knobs to turn. Storing grills, whatever kind, in a shed or garage when not in use is the safest course in preventing an accident.

Ensuring a safe and secure yard is something that needs to be monitored year round. Many people use their yard for different leaving a greater chance of inappropriate and even dangerous items being left in an otherwise safe yard. Continue to monitor the yard for items left and pathways blocked. The yard changes throughout the year and must be attended to on an ongoing basis. Gates must be checked, as should locks from time to time. Certain times of the year, due to extreme heat or cold, it may be prudent to completely deny access to the outdoors without supervision.

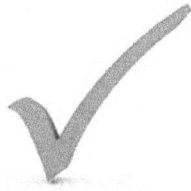

✓ CHAPTER SEVEN CHECKLIST

_____ I have made sure that there's enough light to illuminate pathways.

_____ I have ensured that steps are wide enough and pathways are smooth.

_____If needed, a ramp has been installed in replacement of stairs.

_____All seating areas are comfortable and safe outdoors.

_____I have removed all toys, tools, or items that could be tripped over.

_____I have looked into the plants that are growing in my backyard to ensure they're not toxic.

_____If I have a swimming pool, it has been drained and is covered when not in use.

_____I have stored the barbecue within our locked garage.

_____I have trimmed long twigs, branches, and plants.

CHAPTER EIGHT
FINAL THOUGHTS

You've now taken all the steps you can to ensure that your home will be as safe as possible for someone with Alzheimer's. Prepping your home before your loved one moves in or before the disease progresses will greatly ease your anxiety. Go through those rooms one more time, room-by-room, to assure that you have done all you can to get ready for your loved one to live in your home. Have another family member or friend walk through to spot any potential danger that may have escaped you.

Your safety measures will also reduce stress in the person with Alzheimer's, as the environment will be welcoming, simple, and accommodating to his or her needs. Confusing decisions have already been taken care of by your simplifying the environment, anticipating needs, and altering the surroundings to meet those needs. Dangerous enticements have been altered or removed from sight. The home will be the lesser factor in causing agitation or confusion. You can rest easy as far as the house and its surroundings are concerned.

Remember that you can implement fewer measures in the beginning, if your loved one is still high functioning. Giving greater independence will positively impact your loved one's sense of wellbeing. As long as possible, allow and encourage this independence until changes in your loved one require more restrictive approaches. Add more safety measures as needed.

Despite your work to ensure safety in the home, accidents happen. You can't prevent every risk. Following are some final suggestions to ensure safety beyond home modification.

- **Place STOP, DO NOT ENTER, or CLOSED signs on doors in strategic areas.**

- **Keep shoes, keys, suitcases, coats, hats, and other signs of departure out of sight.**

- **Obtain a medical identification bracelet for the person with Alzheimer's with the words "memory loss" inscribed along with an emergency phone number. Place the bracelet on the person's dominant hand to limit the possibility of removal.**

- **Keep an article of the person's worn, unwashed clothing in a plastic bag to aid in finding someone with the use of dogs.**

- **Notify neighbors of the person's potential to wander or become lost. Alert them to contact you or the police immediately if the individual is seen alone and on the move.**

- **Give local police, neighbors, and relatives a recent photo of the person with Alzheimer's, along with the person's name and pertinent information, as a precaution should he or she become lost. Keep extra photos on hand.**

At some point, despite all the precautionary measures that have been taken, there may come a time when your loved one can no longer stay in your home—or anyone's home. Down the road, care needs may become more than what you can address on your own. Your loved one may require 24-hour care that you cannot provide. Behaviors may have become aggressive, and the individual may be a danger to himself or his caregivers. While a hard decision to make, many families do come to the realization in their journey that their loved one can no longer stay home and needs professional help.

More and more dementia units and certified Alzheimer's units are being opened across the United States. These units go beyond the services of a traditional nursing home as they are established to meet the needs of residents with Alzheimer's or dementia. Staff, trained to deal with the behaviors associated with Alzheimer's disease, provide around-the-clock care.

While many caregivers, particularly family members, resist placing their loved ones out of the home as long as possible, many eventually realize that it is the right decision—for themselves and their loved ones. It is understandable that such a choice would be difficult. Caregivers often feel guilt, as they feel responsible for their loved ones and do not want to let them down.

There is a flip side to this, though, as many individuals respond well to placement in a facility designed to meet their unique needs. Generally, they respond and adjust to their new environment, soon forgetting where they had lived before.

Another benefit to the caregiver comes to passing on the caregiving to professionals. The caregiver no longer has to be the one in charge, the one handling everything. Many spouses, once they relinquish that role, learn to let go and once again enjoy the role of being a wife, husband, or adult child. They can sit and enjoy a visit with their spouse rather than focusing on making meals, putting them to bed, and, yes, changing their diapers. Should this time come, learn to enjoy the freedom as you enter a new phase in your relationship with your loved one.

www.ingramcontent.com/pod-product-compliance
Lightning Source LLC
Chambersburg PA
CBHW080021280326
41934CB00015B/3422